THE EMPTY PICTURE FRAME

An Inconceivable Journey Through Infertility

JENNA CURRIER NADEAU
Contributions by MIKE NADEAU

Outskirts Press, Inc.
Denver, Colorado

Outskirts Press
http://www.outskirtspress.com

ISBN-13: 978-1-4327-0596-1

Library of Congress Control Number: 2007926450

Outskirts Press and the "OP" logo are trademarks belonging to Outskirts Press, Inc.

Printed in the United States of America

To those who struggled yesterday,
those who struggle today,
and those who are struggling to understand.

MTAELA

Table of Contents

Preface
*Just Because You Have a Car,
Doesn't Mean You Know How to Build One*

What has amazed me over the last four years is the ability for every person who learns about our struggle to provide us with the most well intentioned, yet inane advice possible. "Have you tried timing intercourse?" "I've heard yoga can help" and of course the knife in the heart, "If you stop trying, you'll be amazed at how quickly it'll happen. Just relax." No offense to the fertiles of the world, but just because you have a child doesn't mean you have any idea how it got here. I'm sure in your 8th grade science class you learned of fallopian tubes, ovulation, sperm, ovaries, and you might even have been witness to the frightening movie where the mother screams as the baby is being delivered in a horrifying display of excruciating rips and tears. I'm sure you might have even been scared when you heard that a woman could get pregnant anytime, and that's why protection was crucial.

What you probably weren't told was that a fertile couple only has a 20% chance of getting pregnant in any one month, and that more often the window of opportunity isn't 28 days, but closer to 48 hours. You probably missed the part of the lesson that explained how the thickness of the endometrial lining had to be a certain number of millimeters, and that how much fat your body was made of actually played a considerable role in the whole process. The body is a remarkable thing. It can compensate for many imperfections, and for most people it is forgiving of the slightly tilted uterus, or a semi-closed fallopian tube, a weaker quality egg, or a few extra pounds. But for the millions of other women, conceiving a baby is a process that is truly a miracle; a precise combination of old-fashioned faith and the most modern medical technologies.

Infertility is a disease that affects well over six million people in the United States alone. What that statistic fails to consider are the people who are affected by those millions of infertiles; the people who don't know what to say or how to act. These people can't conceive of the inconceivable either, because they have not been faced with infertility or they have not had the desire to raise children. On both sides of the disease are people who feel helpless; unable to fix the problem and incapable of eliminating the pain.

By picking up this book, you are opening a door to the life of an infertile. The journey of my husband and I may not be exactly that of your loved one, but I can assure you the worries, decisions, pain and frustration will be similar. Read these words and you may be able to view your infertile loved one in a new light, and with that light you may understand and empathize with their struggle.

It is my hope that infertiles reading this will find solace in the words of a fellow veteran of this disease. You won't hear me suggest that there is a surefire method to fixing the problem. I don't necessarily believe that in the end everything will work out as it should. What you will hear is my deepest admiration for the path you are on. Perhaps you will find comfort in the words of an infertile couple who has been to hell and back, and has the bruises, both literal and figurative, to prove it.

Introduction

Everyone has them. They are the gifts we receive for a housewarming, or wedding, birthday, or other holiday. They come as silver, gold, wooden, painted, embellished, and engraved. Picture frames. They sit in the closet carefully wrapped in tissue paper until we have just the right photo to match the size and style of the frame.

And then there is the wall. You know the one. The wall in the hallway or in the bedroom, or going up the stairs. It is the showplace for those carefully selected frames. The wall becomes a museum; a place to pay tribute to our loved ones. It is a conversation piece for visitors and a prompt to initiate stories of years ago.

There are delicately selected photos to place in these frames on these walls. Some from long past, of people we may never have met, but whose legacy is firmly carved in our family storyboard. Others, the newest members of our clans, more recent photos, to cover the existing ones, to show the passing of time in steady one-year increments. And still there are others, the most treasured of all; the ones that are neither premeditated nor of time long past. They are the candid photos that capture the essence and spirit of a moment that cannot be retold successfully in a conversation. They are the pictures that truly speak thousands of words.

Empty frames await other things, too. Pressed flowers and birth announcements create shadow boxes filled with memories of the most sacred experiences. Carefully preserved in clay, handprints and footprints forever freeze an age that will never be forgotten. Other frames hold pieces of blankets frayed and faded, once believed to hold magical powers to usurp the demon under a bed or hiding in the closet.

I have these frames, and the walls to hold them. I do not have the pictures or pieces of memorabilia. My frames wait for a day when a tiny, innocent face will smile or laugh in a camera's lens. They are held in a closet for the perfect candid photo of a father adoring his newborn baby and a grandparent sleeping lazily on the couch with a miniaturized version snuggled on top. These photos do not exist. Not yet. And so I have the story, carefully and intricately imagined in my heart. I see black and white photos in these frames, and others containing colorful illustrations of "our family" or handmade Mother's Day cards with lopsided hearts. Today, I see a wall without these memories in a home craving the experiences to capture in those empty frames.

Chapter 1

Children, Children Everywhere,
But Not a One for Me

I was at parent conferences when it happened. A disgruntled mother made the not-so-clever remark, the one I've heard dozens of times in the years I've been teaching 12- and 13-year-olds. Her face contorted, nostrils flared, eyes pierced the distance between us. "Do you have any children of your own?" she questioned spitefully.

My mind was riddled with witty retorts, such as, "I see your child more often and for more hours of the day than you do," and "I have 91 children, thank you." But instead my stomach knotted, a lump in my throat suspended itself and I was certain the angry woman who sat across from me could see it growing out of my turtleneck sweater. I grew cold, numb, and paralyzed by a rhetorical question I've anticipated a number of times. The gravity of my personal failure bubbled to the surface.

"No. No, I do not have children."

1

My husband and I were at our first Neighborhood Walk-Around Christmas Party. We had hesitated to go, as we didn't know anyone, but ultimately thought it was the best way to introduce ourselves to the people who lived in close proximity to ourselves. After all, we had lived there for almost two years and with all of the remodeling that we were doing it, had been difficult to get out and meet people.

Christmas music was playing and a dozen other couples were hovering around a large kitchen island where food was spread out completely covering the granite counters. The, "It's so great to meet you" statement seemed a staple for the evening. Three Coors Lights later and I felt myself relaxing. Everyone was as friendly as they seemed to be when we drove around that first time. We laughed and joked about a rather eccentric neighbor that lives near us. We were fitting in nicely.

Then it happened.

"Do you and your husband have any children?"

In a spilt second, I remembered when we first saw the home we now live in. We drove down the quite road where elementary-aged kids waved at us and mothers were tending to their perfectly landscaped flowerbeds. Dogs raced along their invisible fences as if to chase our car. When the car climbed to the crest of the hill, a small rectangular sign read, "Please drive slowly. We love our children."

This is the perfect neighborhood for our family.

My face began to fall. The carbonation of the beer burned my throat. The reveling sounds of the kitchen blurred into the background as if being pushed down a blackened tunnel.

"No. No, we do not have children."

The exhaust system in my car had a problem. I sat in

the sticky black vinyl chair in the waiting room, pulled out a novel recommended by one of my students, and settled in for the wait. From the corner of my eye, I noted a fellow customer making her way to an empty seat.

"How far along are you?" a voice pops out from behind the cashier's window.

Don't look up. You don't want to see this.

"I'm due on May." The woman sat next to me.

Oh God, definitely don't look up.

"Me too, I'm due on May 2nd," replied the receptionist.

Me too. Once. But not anymore. No, not anymore.

I was at my six-month teeth cleaning appointment; an appointment that I usually put off until I'm two or three months past due. I waited impatiently for the whole thing to be over with. *I never get out of here with good news. Why would this time be different? Maybe I've run out of teeth to have cavities on. No, then they'd just start replacing them.* When my name was called, a hygienist that I had never met before greeted me. She was bubbly and welcoming. *Not a bad start. Let's give this one a shot, shall we?*

I sank into the faux leather reclining chair while she wrapped the paper bib around my neck and began making polite conversation. *This is going to be sort of a one-sided conversation, lady. I can't really offer any feedback with a mouthful of your fingers and metal utensils.*

"So, how's the little one doing?" *You didn't just say that.*

"What?" *I must have heard wrong.*

"The baby?"

"Um, I don't have a baby." *Smile, laugh politely... it's not her fault. She's got the wrong person. Maybe she thinks you're your sister. She's new; easy mistake.*

"Yes you do. You are Jenna Nadeau right? Did I call

3

the wrong person in?"

"I'm Jenna, but I don't have a baby."

"Sure you do." *I think I'd know if I had a baby.* "I swear I just read it in your chart."

"I don't have a baby. I promise you that." *Just clean my teeth, would you?*

"Oh dear, I can't let this go. Let me see what I was looking at... Yep, here it is. Last October you declined the x-rays because you said you were pregnant. What happened?" *What do you think happened?*

"I lost him."

Silence.

"Oh my. Well, I'm sure you'll have another one in no time at all. When it's meant to be."

And of course there was Oprah. I sat on her butter crème colored couch prepared to talk about what it was like to be in my 30's and struggling with infertility. It was the first interview on the topic that I had seen on television, and I didn't want to blow it. I had dreams of representing women everywhere who felt scared, lonely and exhausted by the trials of infertility and didn't have a voice in our society. A few questions into the interview, Oprah asked me if I had made peace with being infertile. The "loss of a dream," as she says. I hadn't thought of it that way. I didn't think I had actually "lost" my dream. I guess, even after over four years, two IUI's, four IVF's, two FET's and one miscarriage, I still was hopeful. While I had entertained the thought of not having a biological child, I certainly never considered that I wouldn't be a mom. I only thought my dream to be postponed. But lost? Me? No, not me.

It's everywhere all the time. Thoughts of the children we don't have or the ones we have lost are constantly in our thoughts. Infertility is inescapable. Whether we are shopping at the mall, surrounded by loving family and friends at holidays or celebrations, or watching infomercials late at night, baby thoughts are everywhere.

As young girls we are handed dolls that mimic babies. They poop, pee, need to be burped, and cry. We take care of them; changing diapers, brushing their hair, and walking them down the street in strollers. Before we hit puberty we have the names of our children selected, and the most popular job for a young girl seems to be babysitting our neighbors' young ones. So young we were and already we were caregivers, preparing for the role of motherhood.

The world is unforgiving to infertiles. History teaches of women who were beheaded for their inability to reproduce, and let's face it, it is the ability, not the choice, to bear children that is the primary physical difference between men and women. So, where does that put me? Where does that put the millions of women who have not been given the choice of having children? The painful struggle to conceive and maintain a pregnancy is one of the few remaining taboo topics in a society that freely debates over varying lifestyles, abortion rights, disease and warfare.

Maybe you are dealing with infertility. Maybe it's someone you love. Either way, it's not an easy disease to understand. From the outside, you can research as I did; spend hours and hours on the internet or in a library, or calling doctors, just to find out a bunch of facts and figures. But infertility isn't a disease of statistics and to limit the conversation to what medications will produce which results, and which tests should be performed, minimizes the toll it can take on the individual. This isn't a resource book that will overwhelm the reader with a lot of medical jargon, tests or alternative cures. That's what the doctors are for. I'm not a doctor; I'm a patient. My expertise is from the inside; the body, the heart, and the soul of the infertile.

When infertility is discussed in the books I've thumbed through, the intent seems to be to lighten the topic and reduce it to punch lines and silly anecdotes. My journey wasn't fun and it wasn't funny. Sure, having a sense of humor about the devastation of infertility is not just important, but necessary in order to maintain some semblance of normalcy in public life. Anyone who knows me will attest to the streaming sarcasm that spewed from my mouth or the self-deprecating humor that helped me put a spin on the difficult times. But, more often then I laughed, I cried. I cried and cried some more. I cried because of what I lost; I cried for what I never had. I cried because I wanted to be understood and I cried because I wanted to be left alone. This isn't easy, but not many diseases are. It is a disease that affects every person associated with the infertile. This disease is as personal as it gets, and as misunderstood as they come.

This is the story of love, loss, lessons and the infertile.

Chapter 2

We Did Everything Right.
What Could Go Wrong?

We had been together for years before we got married. Six to be exact. I was 20, and he was 21 when Mike and I met. Living side-by-side in a duplex in the middle of nowhere, New Hampshire during our senior year of college can make even enemies come together, and we certainly were far from that. From the moment I met him, we connected. It wasn't romantic at first; the typical college experience of parties, work, more parties and figuring out if there really was life after college. It was an exciting time for both of us, and somehow through all of the chaos and confusion, we managed to find each other. Talk about opposites attracting. Mike was, and is, one of the nice guys. I was the girl who was perpetually attracted to the bad boy. If there was an easy way, I took the hard way. If there was an opportunity to challenge his point of view, I jumped right on it. He pulled and I pushed. He was often passive and calm, while I was passionate and unwavering. I found him intriguing. He wasn't rough on the edges and he didn't want to impress anyone with rebellious actions or the need to brag in order to get attention.

Mike would cross the threshold from his side of the duplex to mine and night after night we would hang out in my room, listening to music, talking about our families, and trying to decide what to do with our lives. Conversations were easy and before we knew it, 7 p.m. turned into 3 a.m. and we would fall asleep in the middle of a thought. He was a friend, someone who made me laugh every day and challenged me to dream bigger than I thought I deserved. Before knowing Mike, I accepted what I considered to be a reasonable amount of failure, never thinking I could, and should, be striving for more. In the first months of our friendship, I was already a better person; more ambitious about my future and more accepting of my past transgressions. We grew together without even realizing it, and suddenly found that our friendship had evolved into a love for each other that was deep, respectful and unconditional.

Shortly after we graduated, I began working towards my master's degree and started a full year internship teaching 8th grade language arts. I adored children and from the early days of babysitting, I knew that any career I would have would need to involve kids. The hours were long. Exhaustion set in by the end of the first week. I quickly found that not a day would go by without one of us, my students or myself, falling to tears. It was a challenge I sometimes questioned, and yet all the while Mike was there to push me along and give me the confidence to pursue both my degree and my career with all of the effort I could command.

If salary was indicative of commitment, we would have

8

had it made. Unfortunately, making $26,000 a year in the beginning was not going to be enough to build the life Mike and I began talking about. But being a teacher was never about making money. It was a difficult time, trying to reconcile a career dream with the possibility that this choice could inhibit my other dreams from being realized. Mike, however, was sure we could have it all, and he found a way to make certain I never had to compromise my career for my other ambitions.

At 22 and 23, with our eyes fixed on getting ahead of the financial game early in life, we purchased an old Victorian house in a small town near the university from which we had graduated. Together with another friend, we renovated the old dilapidated house and turned it into a rental property. A great investment, yes, but not without its shortcomings. For the first time, we had moved in together, but the circumstances were far from ideal. We found ourselves living on the same side of a duplex; a one-bathroom, run down, flea-infested apartment that needed more than the coat of paint we had envisioned. While renting out one side, we renovated the near uninhabitable apartment.

There was a period of five weeks where we took daily showers at the gym down the road and used the corner gas station or buckets for toilets while reconstruction was underway. Each night, after work, we were painting, cleaning, rewiring, and building. While other people our age were still in the stage of partying and finding employment, Mike and I were already working towards a goal of being financially independent. We had larger ideals in mind; to marry, build a family and not be faced with the stresses of money that can affect so many young couples. As passionate as I was about the students I taught, Mike was equally invested in his work as a man of finance and business. It was important to him that we protected ourselves and controlled as many of the variables as was possible. We were making progress. We were making the right choices and with each sacrificed night of pouring sweat equity into that property, we knew we were on our way.

Combining the income of the rental property with the money we were making through our first years in the working world, we were able to expand our dreams of adulthood into purchasing a small condo where we could begin a more permanent relationship. We sold the old Victorian house that same year and the gamble paid off. We were able to establish a safety net for ourselves unlike anything we would have been otherwise capable of amassing. At 26 and 27 years old, we had achieved the first of many goals that was once discussed during those late night conversations in college.

A word from Mike…

If there is one thing I know in this world, it is finance. I received the majority of my training from my dad. I guess you could say I really like money and even before I graduated high school I fully expected to be rich by the age of thirty. I started my financial adventure quite early in life. Admittedly, I was quite proud of myself. As soon as I got out of college, I knew it was time to stop paying rent to a landlord. Since I didn't have much money, I convinced my best friend and girlfriend at the time (Jenna) to purchase a multi-family house. It was a great time in the housing market and we got a great deal. I was 25 years old and on my way to financial freedom.

Not many people our ages could say they were taking steps forward like that. It might have been risky to some,

---

but for me it was one of the best moves we could all have made. I had to pat myself on the back for this major move. I knew I didn't want to be a slave to my job when I was 60, nor did I want to be struggling to finance college tuitions for my children. I wanted it all and I was hungry to take steps in the right direction.

Jenna was a huge part of that 'right direction'. She was passionate and faithful to her values. She was an amazingly loyal friend and as supportive of a girlfriend as I could have imagined. She hung in with me when I wanted to take business risks with the rental property, and her belief in me was what made it a success.

One of the many reasons I fell in love with Mike was because of his ambition. I was amazed at what was possible when he was around. He had dreams that required intense commitment and a vision for our life that was remarkable. I don't think we realized we were in the midst of a tremendous love story.

Six years after meeting, Mike proposed. We had a modest one-bedroom condo and two cats. We had established our careers, bonded our families, and put money away in a savings account. Mike and I had seen each other through six years of turbulent experiences, from the loss of loved ones, the fears and anxieties of our first years of working, to the uncertainty of our entrepreneurial endeavor with the investment property. When we said our vows on that cold December day in New England, it was with open eyes and a genuine love and admiration for each other.

Chapter 3

Even Though You Build it,
They Don't Always Come

Like most newly married couples, we were ready to start the rest of our lives. We had been together for many years and had been the closest of friends, business partners, and now, spouses. It was time to begin working on a family. We purchased a home in a beautiful neighborhood and began envisioning a Christmas tree in the family room with kids climbing over us to unwrap presents. I dreamed of birthdays, kindergarten and other milestones in our life together with children. We were building a life that was uniquely ours and I was entirely proud of every step. I had never had such a feeling of confidence that each decision we had made was leading up to the experience of starting our family.

A word from Mike:

When Jenna and I purchased our first house as a

married couple, she concentrated on the decorating and I immediately started putting every extra penny towards the principle in order to pay down the mortgage each month. Jenna made it a home and I made sure it was a home we could afford. Just like in the days of the rental property, we both brought our talents to the table. We were a great team.

We were both putting a significant amount of our salaries into our retirement plans. I was working my tail off at my job to move ahead quickly and make a name for myself. Things were falling into place nicely. Hard work was paying off and the profits from our financial plans were going to pay off in spades. I felt in total control of our future. We would have the house paid off within eight years under the payment plan I had us on.

Although we had been together for a long time, we were still very different in many ways. I liked to take chances and throw myself into situations. I was driven by emotion and passion. Mike was much more methodical. It had taken him six years to propose, not because he was unsure of our commitment, but because he was never very comfortable with change unless he had worked out every possible angle, good and bad.

Mike wanted a family, but he wanted to take things slowly. He was afraid that, having just gotten married, we needed time to settle into a new routine before introducing a baby to the program. We had many conversations about this and eventually decided that we would start taking steps to ensure my body was ready for pregnancy. I was going to stop taking my birth control, begin eating healthier, and taking better care of myself physically. In the meantime, we would leave conception up to fate and not actively try to have a baby for a few months.

Step one was to stop the birth control pills I had been on since my late teen years. I had started taking them because, unlike all of my girlfriends, I was seventeen and still had never had a period. I suppose this should have been a giant red flag waving in my face for years, but during that time it was more of a blessing than a curse. My doctor at the time told me that taking the pill would be a way to regulate me. It did. Each month I got a period and for the next ten years I faithfully took cycle after cycle with the greatest faith that I was as normal as the next woman.

But after three months of not being on the pill and not seeing a period, I went to a doctor. She insisted that being irregular was common in women who stopped the pill. I felt strongly that this was not the typical situation. My history of never having my period left me feeling uneasy about the "wait and see" approach. Nonetheless, who was I to question a doctor? I waited. I waited months and months, until we were six months into waiting, and when I still had not had a period, I called the doctor again. She assured me that this was normal for some women, but that a magic pill called Provera, when taken for five days, would bring on a period and things would probably be back to normal. She was right… and wrong. The first time I took it, it worked just fine, a one-day period, but it was still a period, so I felt successful. Then, one month I took the five pills and I waited the 10 days, but not a single sign of a period came.

Monday, July 7, 2003
MISSING - REWARD OFFERED

Okay, seriously, can ANYTHING go right with my body? The ten days are up and still no sign of my period. Nothing, nada, totally MIA.

I've spent the entire week sitting on the couch researching what could be wrong with me and how I can make it right. The only thing I came up with was parsley... so of course I've been drinking cup after cup of the stuff and even though I seem to get a faint spot here and there, the doctor's office won't consider it to be "the real thing"... URGHHH, this is unbelievable. "The Real Thing" is completely laughable. I've never had the REAL thing... just some fake substitute. The more I don't get my period, the more nervous, anxious and frustrated I become, and that isn't helping anything.

This is where the balloons and confetti should appear from the ceiling, because Jenna's pity party is about to begin...

I just don't understand this. We've been doing this for months now, and every time I feel like we are a step closer to becoming pregnant, something pulls the rug from under me. Even the basics aren't working. The Provera was supposed to fix this. I didn't really expect it to fix everything and make me normal again, but I did think it would give me a temporary period. Now, not even that is effective, which means I may have to try a whole month of birth control pills just to get a period. Here I go again... back to the old standby. Mike and I are ready to start having kids and we are reverting back to birth control. How is that ever going to help conceive a baby?

I'm starting to feel like this is going to be a long road. I know it's only been a few months, but there is a whisper constantly in my heart that I need to settle into a more patient place. It may be a very bumpy road.

I took it again. This time ten pills and I waited 14 days. Lo and behold, I got a period that lasted for about 36 hours. At least it was something. Things returned to normal; just normal for me, not for the rest of the women I knew. More months went by and my doctor told me to see a nutritionist. I was 105 pounds and 5'4". She was convinced that a few pounds would make all the different for me. In the meantime, I was to take my temperature, commonly known as Basal Body Temperature (BBT), each morning to determine when I ovulated.

I saw the nutritionist and in one month I managed to increase my weight to 112 pounds, enough to get my Body Mass Index (BMI) to the middle range of average for my height. Still no period. More Provera for the "kick-start", and still no kick-start. Months into faithfully trying to conceive had amounted to months of realizing this was going to be tougher than we had thought. Taking my temperature each morning became a monotonous act in futility. There was not a rise and fall pattern like I had seen on the example charts. I bought three of those thermometers, thinking they were broken, and I faithfully kept them under my pillow so I could take my resting temperature with the least possible movement. Still, my chart looked like the toothed edge of a saw. My next doctor's appointment would confirm what I was already suspecting; I hadn't ovulated. In fact, I had NEVER ovulated. All of those years of being on the pill and in all the years prior to that, never had my body released a single egg; I never had a shot.

This was a defining moment for me, because in all of the years prior to this revelation, I had trusted my doctors. I believed they were not just doing what was right for the moment, but that they were actually fixing my problem. My problem was that I didn't get my period, and with the pill, I did. Problem solved, right? Not exactly. For the ten years that I was taking that medication, my body, a reproductive system that had never functioned correctly, was essentially put to sleep. My ovaries were suppressed to not ovulate, while the issue of why I hadn't ovulated was never actually explored.

I felt cheated. I felt abandoned. I had taken for granted that my body was just going to do what it was supposed to do. A decision was made in my mind that I would never blindly trust information that was given to me regardless of whom it came from or how many degrees were framed on their walls. This moment was the beginning of me taking control of my body, but it was not the end of the problems.

We had passed the year mark quickly and the situation was beginning to take its toll. For the past several years, things always had a way of falling into place. Why would this be any different? We were prepared for children in so many ways. We had saved money. We were educated people with good jobs, and we had a fantastic family who supported us and would welcome a baby at any time.

Our friends had started to build families of their own. Of the five couples we were closest to, three of them were pregnant already. Dreams of our children growing up together weighed on my mind. I hadn't realized how fully engrained the picture of my future was in my heart. I felt pressure of my own making and I knew that wasn't making it easier for my body to do what it had never done before. I was disappointed, but I wasn't defeated. I knew there were more strategies, other medications, and we weren't ready to throw in the towel.

Clomiphene citrate (Clomid) was next on the menu. Another little white pill that, when taken for a few days, would most certainly allow me to ovulate. This seemed to be the answer I was looking for. I had read medical articles and listened to my doctor tell me that sometimes all it takes is to ovulate once and the body will recognize the process and adapt to it regularly. This was the first real "infertility treatment" that I had experienced and the first time I had heard someone actually use the word "infertility" in my presence. Up until now, I only had "trouble conceiving."

Monday, August 2, 2004

Watching the Wheels Go Round and Round

There's a great John Lennon song, "Watching the Wheels." There was a time when I felt like that was me; relaxed, "Just sittin here watching the wheels go round and round, I really love to watch them roll"... I listen to that song and remember the times in college when the most stressful thing about my life was how I was going to get off the couch to order some chicken fingers and fries from Pizza Spinners. I loved those days when responsibility was secondary to having fun and enjoying the friends around me.

I guess that's still me to some extent, except that I've been watching myself spin wheels for 1.7 years and I'm dizzy, irritable, and really want to get off of this ride. This merry-go-round is no fun at all. Each month is the same... a fresh start, a clean slate, and every hope in the world that in 28 days Mike and I will get the news that we are going to be the latest couple to move to parenthood. I guess that is my first problem...

Twenty-eight days? Where did I come up with that number? Oh yeah, that's the cycle length of a normal person. Not me... I'm rare, unique, one of a kind. My cycles? Well, My first cycle was 27 years long. But thanks to Clomid that's about to end.

There are so many ways that this whole adventure could turn out and I have every reason to believe that my worries and frustrations are just the dramatics of being Jenna. I haven't been known for my patience and when there was an opportunity to make a small issue into a larger concern, I was there to build my emotions until I had convinced myself that there was something really wrong with me. I could turn a headache into a brain tumor and convince myself that a common cold was the beginning of full blow pneumonia.

Taking a pill in this situation is a perfectly doable and

appropriate course of action. It makes sense; it's just not that aggressive. Not aggressive enough for having tried for this long. What do I want to be doing? I don't know. I don't know anything about this. That's probably a good thing. If I knew of the possibilities, I'd be convincing myself that I was dying or something equally tragic.

But I keep hanging in there, thinking that if I just go with the flow, things will work out. And so here I am, about to take my little white pills, watching the wheels spinning round and round, hoping that one day they will stop and I'll be able to jump on the next ride: motherhood.

I found some wonderful articles on some reputable websites and I felt encouraged by an online message board where women were talking about not just ovulating, but ovulating multiple eggs at once while on this medication. They wrote of taking over-the-counter cold expectorants as a way to increase cervical fluid, which would facilitate sperm to reach the egg. I took it. I also consumed green tea in mass quantities for the same purpose. I was reading terms like "egg white cervical mucus" and was daunted by disc-like contraptions that resembled diaphragms to keep the sperm inside for a longer period of time. These ladies wrote of special lubricants and ideal sexual positions for conception. Some of them were using actual egg whites to facilitate sperm transportation. Okay, this seemed odd to say the least, and I never quite got myself to try that one, but some of these women swore by it. Who was I to judge? Anything seemed better than the 'wait and see' method I had been subscribing to. The more I delved into these buddy boards, the more certain I was that this was going to be the answer to our prayers. These women were such an incredible wealth of knowledge. It was like I had discovered a hidden society of people who were just like

19

me. I had luckily stumbled into a club of ladies with the secret decoder ring for infertility. With some well-timed intercourse, we would have our family. I was convinced of that. To some degree I was even concerned with the possibility of having twins.

Three months of Clomid and on the first cycle, I ovulated for the very first time. I felt strangely like I was finally a woman. Something that the kids I taught were starting to do on their own, naturally, and here I was, at 29 years old, and for the first time my body had functioned. There was so much hope for us. Right on time, Mike and I did the whole procreation dance thing. With my hips propped up on pillows and laying still for a strong hour afterwards, I thought for sure we had hit the jackpot.

We had crested a hill and reached a moment of possibility. I was ovulating for the first time in my life and now, thanks to a mixture of modern medicine, and old wives tales, I was even going to have the opportunity to become pregnant. A little pill was easy to take and even though I had learned that it's not usually given for more than six cycles, I was confident that we needed only a couple to call an end to the problem.

Sadly, that first cycle ended in failure. We knew that was a possibility, but it seemed that if I could ovulate, the rest would happen as it did for the people around us. It didn't, and two more Clomid cycles would fare even worse. Not only was I not pregnant, but my body stopped responding to the medication even when the dose was increased. Once again, I hadn't ovulated. Once again, there was no opportunity for us to be pregnant.

A word from Mike:

After we got married, I could tell that Jenna was ready to have children right away. I wanted to just take it slow and get used to being married. I'm sure many guys can understand where I'm coming from. I thought I was too immature and in spite of all of the financial preparations, I didn't think we were ready to introduce a child into this world.

Once it was time to start to grow our family, I'll admit I still wasn't fully ready. I have never known of any infertility issues in my family, so I was confident that it would be clear sailing once we started. My mom once told me that she got pregnant with my twin sister, Kelly, and me within a few months of trying to conceive. My grandparents had a total of eight children with no signs of infertility problems. Jenna's parents were each one of four kids. Having babies was not a problem in either of our families.

The day Jenna and I had the conversation about coming off the pill scared the hell out of me. I even tried to avoid the discussion entirely. In my mind, this meant I'd be a father in nine months. I don't know about other people, but it takes me time to adapt to change.

I became very surprised when Jenna wasn't pregnant after trying naturally for about six months. I could sense she was becoming increasingly uneasy and anxious. I tried to tell her that everything was alright, but it didn't make her feel any better. She would say things like, "You don't understand." She was right. It wouldn't be far from the realm of possibility for her to get worked up about something. I just didn't think it was big deal. Over the next few months, Jenna started taking Clomid. I was pretty confident with the introduction of this drug that our chances were now 200%. I was just waiting for the news that she was pregnant. Month after month though, we continued to get disappointing news.

It didn't take more than a few rounds of Clomid to heighten my own anxieties about the situation. I still thought we would be pregnant in no time at all, but there was a small question mark forming in my head. I tried to keep my head together and be the voice of calm, but truthfully, I was starting to understand the nervousness Jenna was experiencing.

Then came the news I had really not prepared myself for. Following the last Clomid cycle, I met with my OB/GYN to discuss what the next course of action could be. I assumed there was some other kind of pill or maybe a combination of medications to try. Instead, I was told, "It's time to pull out the big guns, Jenna. I am sending you to a reproductive endocrinologist."

By this time, nearly two years had passed and we were walking into uncharted territory. All couples in our circle of friends were pregnant or had already given birth. I felt like an outsider; like the kid who gets kicked off the lunch table and pretends they are sick so they can go to the nurse's office instead of sitting alone in humiliation. Outside of the cyber women whose circles I lurked in, I did not know a single person who had experienced what I was about to. The closest people in my life, with whom I had grown up with through grade school and on to college, began to feel like strangers. This was the first time I felt alone in our struggle. Then we learned the news that would change our lives completely.

Our medical insurance was not going to cover any of the treatments that I might need to fix whatever this problem was. How could that be? We both had great jobs and we had paid considerably for a fantastic policy. This was when I realized that apparently, only a handful of states in our country mandated this kind of coverage and ours wasn't one of them. At the date of this writing there are only 15 states in our country which mandate medical insurance coverage to carry in their policy a provision for infertility. These states are: Arkansas, California, Connecticut, Hawaii, Illinois, Louisiana, Maryland, Massachusetts, Montana, New Jersey, New York, Ohio, Rhode Island, Texas and West Virginia. We live in New Hampshire where there is no such law. No matter how good our policies are, or what we do for a living, in New Hampshire, a person with infertility issues is on their own to bear the weight of the financial burden.

Our plans were on hold. Our family was not going to expand. We couldn't go any further. We had positioned ourselves for the life we believed we were meant for. Our beautiful four-bedroom home, our family friendly cars, even my job as a teacher, and here we were facing the possibility that it was all in vain.

The one thing we knew was that going into debt was not an option. We had spent too much time working on building a solid foundation for our lives and we weren't ready to start writing checks. Instead, we researched for months to be sure we had found a proper doctor and we had compiled a list of questions and concerns to present at our consultation. In the meantime, we saved money.

I took on a part-time job teaching summer school and coaching some extracurricular sports at school. Mike was already working late hours, but added a side job painting a coworker's newly remodeled house. We began a budget that saved us nickels and dimes. These dimes led to quarters and dollars. Before we knew it, we were on our way to paying for some of the fees associated with seeing a reproductive endocrinologist (RE).

The money we saved helped us to begin the initial testing and procedures at our infertility clinic. Also, our insurance company agreed to pay for what they considered diagnostic work: blood tests and Mike's sperm analysis. This was a fortunate break, but we realized the need to dip into our savings account anyway, the "emergency fund", so that we could proceed with a hysterosalpingogram (HSG), a procedure where the doctor used a dye in the fallopian tubes to rule out structural anomalies.

I had done some reading about this procedure and from what I understood, I could expect it to be similar to a pelvic exam; simple and painless. I read post after post on the internet about this and they all seemed the same. I had no concerns for anything but a slight distortion of my pride as I lay on the table, legs wide open for a handful of doctors. Unfortunately, this was the first shock I had. It was my first hideous introduction to the world of infertility.

Like I said, most people I had encountered had no trouble at all with this procedure. Maybe, in retrospect, it was more tolerable than I had believed, but in the moments that I was on the table, I couldn't imagine anything worse. The RE was saying things like, "Just a small cramp here." *Are you kidding?* I was grasping the sides of the table and my fingers were digging into the paper liner beneath me. "Okay, Jenna, you've got a bit of a tilted uterus here, so this might be a little awkward." *Awkward? Farting in a public place is awkward. This is far from awkward.* "Now try to relax, this is just going to pinch a bit." *Pinch?* With those words I felt what can only be described as the stepping on a tack barefooted. I immediately began to cry. A nurse came to my side and started rubbing my forehead and holding my hand. "Oh, that wasn't that bad." *Yeah, maybe not for you, but then again you aren't lying on this table with you legs in stirrups and your crotch exposed to*

bunch of strangers. And there's that other little matter...
you aren't a WOMAN!!! But sure, it wasn't that bad.

This test produced normal results; no blockages to speak of. Structurally, it appeared that I was in fine condition. I was diagnosed with hypothalamic amenorrhea, a condition for which there wasn't a cure, but there were things that could be done in order to have my body function long enough to produce a baby. It was there that we focused our attention.

Mike and I were making a good living and by the grace of God we had made some smart financial moves early into our relationship. We had amassed the suggested six to eight months of savings and while this procedure and its prerequisite testing would take a bit of a chunk from that, we felt confident that it was there for a reason and building a family was as good an emergency as any. We decided to see this as an investment instead of a bill, and with the greatest amount of optimism we could muster, we handed over approximately $3,000, not including the additional $500 for medication. Thirty-five hundred dollars was a hefty bill for one month, but it was only going to be one month, right? This money allowed us to begin our first round of artificial treatment known as intrauterine insemination (IUI).

Monday, February 14, 2005
It Ain't Just Flowers and Candy Anymore

It's Valentine's Day and we just got back from the clinic for our class on injections. I would never have thought this would be my idea of a romantic experience, yet in all the years of flowers, dinners, and jewelry, this was undoubtedly, the best Valentine's

Day experience.

I admit this was an intimidating time for both of us. I felt overwhelmed sitting in the office surrounded by five other women who were all after the same thing. I looked around and realized that statistically, one, at the most of us, would find something to smile about by the end of the first cycle. But Mike sat next to me, and together we absorbed as much as we could, scribbling notes, asking questions, and holding hands. With only one other man in the class, I had to smile to myself that I was fortunate to have my husband there, knowing that these other women were going to be doing this alone or would have to try and explain this immense about of information to their husbands later. Mike took the afternoon off from work so that he could be there with me and be a part of the introduction to injections. The nurse passed around needles and showed us how to keep everything organized. She acted like it was no big deal at all and as much as I'd love to have that kind of ambivalence to the whole thing, I don't ever want to become that accustomed to this process.

It was such a tremendous relief to have him there. I had originally said that I could just do the class on my own, but when I sat there and tried to soak it in, I knew I didn't just want him there, I needed him there.

When the time comes, I can do the shots myself. But Mike decided he wants to be a part of it. I'm glad for that; it will take a bit of the pressure off of me to make this all happen. For now, the meds are ordered and all we need to do is wait for the Provera to kick in. Tonight is my last pill, so if all goes according to plan, we should be starting the injections next week. Of course, as I type this, I realize how ridiculous "all goes according to plan" sounds... Hell, if all went according to plan, I'd be working on baby number two by now!

Oh well, we can hope, can't we?

Of course, it wouldn't be quite as easy as popping the Provera and waiting a few days. Time passed slowly while we sat around waiting to begin. All of the medications were lined up on the bathroom counter and I had read through the two-inch binder of material provided by the clinic. I had practiced twisting the needles onto the syringes half a dozen times. I even reverted to my old behaviors of drinking parsley tea by the quart, even though that had never proven to do the trick before.

Wednesday, March 2, 2005
Let the Games Begin

It's been two weeks since the Provera and, of course, it wasn't the simple process of taking a few pills, but finally, yesterday morning I woke up to my period. This morning I officially started the IUI process with my day 2 blood work and ultrasound. It was so exciting to go into the clinic and know that we were on our way after so much time... We are really going to have a baby this time!

I was trying hard all day at school to keep my mind off of the phone call that should have been on my machine when I got home. I didn't want to get my hopes up, but I was confident that they would be giving us the instructions for what we should be doing next.

Sure enough, the woman on the machine told us that we could start our injections on Friday and continue them through the weekend. On Monday I will go back in to have blood work done and see where we are at. The nurses have explained all of this to us; the cycle, the shots, the actual insemination, but here we are at the cusp of everything and the knot is my stomach is indescribable.

My mind is racing with promise and excitement now. There is so much for us to look forward to and even though we've felt this

27

way before when we did the Clomid, HSG, sperm analysis and the other tests, this time feels different. I know this is a huge step for us, financially and emotionally. But in a year from now when I am watching Mike hold our baby(ies), there is no price I wouldn't have paid. My mind is afraid of the disappointment. I know our chances even with this are just as good as a normal person; 20%, but that's 20% more chance than I've ever had before. My heart just wants, no needs, to feel some sense of possibility. We haven't had that in so long.

Cycling for the IUI produced a lot of long days. I would come home from school and spend hour upon hour searching the internet and reading books–everything from the medication I was taking to the possible symptoms I could expect to feel if I were pregnant. I'm sure to some people that would sound obsessive. To me it was the only part of the conception process over which I could have some semblance of control.

I was a mixture of emotions. I felt like we were making progress on the road that would soon lead to pregnancy. My spirits were high, but so were my fears. Despite my researching and preparation, I hadn't done this before, and each new test result sent me into moments of tremendous excitement or intense worry. I fully believed the IUI process would work for us. I fully believed we had solved the problem of not ovulating. I even pictured tucking in our babies at night, and when I closed my eyes I could smell them in the "cute baby from the bathtub" way. At the same time, I was afraid to let myself fully experience all of these emotions and often I would stop them before a complete smile formed on my face. It had been over two years since we began trying to have a family and two years of disappointments caused paper cuts in the daydreams.

28

Wednesday, March 9, 2005
Disappointment... Deja vu or a premonition?

In the last eight days I've amazed myself with how good I am at giving myself shots. This is not a fun time, but Mike and I are making our way through it. It could be a lot worse. Promptly at 8 p.m. each night we go into the master bathroom and while he is dialing up our dosage, I'm doing the alcohol swab thing on the little fat sack I've created around my belly button. We've got a nice little system going now. Strangely, this might actually bring us closer together.

This morning I had my day 10 blood work and ultrasound. I went in thinking I was going to get some great news. Everything seemed to be in my favor. The fact that they had kept me on 37.5 units of the medication for the last two days confirmed in my head that I was responding well to the meds. It's a low dose; as low as it goes, and for me to respond to any meds is a great thing all by itself. Of course, I should have known by the crappy weather and the fact that I was getting super sick that this was not going to be my day.

Our doctor was in the room while the ultrasound was being done and that made me excited... again, thinking I'd be taking the "trigger shot" soon and that we might have the IUI this weekend. As soon as the numbers started coming up, I realized how stupid my excitement was.

I have a bunch of small follicles that don't even get to be measurable, and only one that amounted to over the minimum... it's 10.1mm... miserable. As if that punch in the gut wasn't enough, the endometrial lining was 4.3mm... truly pathetic and not even enough to support a flea. I tried so hard to joke it off and be sarcastic, but my eyes were filling up and the doctor knew I was really upset.

I don't know what to think now. Mike was really good about the news. He hugged me and told me to wait for the clinic to call and tell me what we do next. I know that I'm not the first person to be in this situation. I know that other women have gotten pregnant with much worse circumstances. But none of that matters right now. I'm not other women and I don't want their worse circumstances.

Right now all I can think about is the fact that I've felt this disappointment every month for two years. And what's worse than the deja vu is the idea that this isn't a feeling reserved for the past. I feel like it's an all too familiar feeling preparing me for the future.

Ugh, I hate that. I hate that there I am, preparing myself for a heartache before it's happened. I started out so positive and I had every intention to continue that. I have to stop this right now... it's too easy to go from happy to sad, and far too difficult to go in the reverse direction. I CAN DO THIS!!! I AM GOING TO BE PREGNANT!!! Get it together Jenna. Get in the game or go home. There can be no more of this flip-flopping nonsense.

In the day that followed, I decided that I couldn't spend each moment wrapped up in the process and that I would need to believe it was positive in order for it to turn out successfully. The difficulty was opening myself up to envisioning everything I had wanted for so long. To make myself vulnerable to the possibility of a cycle working in our favor meant I had to let my guard down long enough to welcome the dreams. This was a tall order for someone who had lived many years in defense of potential calamity. It had taken a lot of energy to be in a constant state of worry and I was exhausted from the negativity. Far more than that, however, I was scared of the crush of defeat. In my mind, I equated allowing myself to feel optimistic with setting myself up for a freefall of disappointment.

I did my very best. When a glimmer of pessimism surfaced, I would push it away with daydreams of baby showers, nightly feedings, soccer games, and teenage temper tantrums. I took the bits of negative energy and lack of confidence and turned them into gratitude for the opportunity to be able to go through the process that would gain us the family Mike and I had prayed for.

Sunday, March 13, 2005

Every Cloud Has a Silver Lining

Yesterday I got word that Pepe had passed away. It's been a long winter waiting for this eventuality, but now that it's here, I'm not ready to grasp it completely. We've heard the "24-48 hours" so many times, that I feel like we were living in a perpetual state of limbo.

I'm not sure how to feel now. I am sad and overwhelmed with the loss of my last grandparent, and yet I feel a sense of relief that my family can move forward with living instead of being on the verge of the steady decline towards death. I have memories of Nana's death and the impact that had on my father. I worry for him.

Still another part of me is feeling more confident about our own baby now that there is one more person in heaven looking over us. Is that entirely selfish? I had another round of blood work and ultrasound today, and learned that I have two "dominant follicles", 14.3mm and 13.7mm, and that my lining is at a comfortable 7.6. Thank you Estrace suppositories! Tonight I will do another shot of the Follistim and go back for blood work tomorrow. My arm is feeling sore and is slightly bruised, but I keep telling myself that this is well worth it. This is a minor annoyance by comparison to what we've already been through. I feel like this is the moment I've been waiting for and that the inseminations are just around the corner.

I'm scared, nervous, and excited, and hoping that this will be the last time I will need to feel this way. I'm praying that Pepe, Nana, and all of the other people I love are watching over us and holding my hand for the moment that I have wanted so much to happen. I can't wait for the inseminations. I can't wait for our prayers to become our reality!

Conceiving a baby had stopped being a romantic notion long before this IUI cycle. From timing intercourse to the daily conversations about doctor appointments and sperm analysis results, I held no naïve notions that our child would be conceived in a log cabin with snow falling gently outside. There were to be neither candles nor soft music. Truthfully, I wasn't that kind of person anyway. But I definitely didn't picture the cold room and the bright fluorescent lights of an exam table. And the lady standing at the business end of the stirrups with a long catheter containing Mike's washed and separated sperm was far from my imagination.

Nonetheless, there we were. We arrived at the clinic early, probably due to the anticipation and excitement of the day. Mike was immediately taken to a back room where he gave his "sample".

A word from Mike:

I think most men probably joke about going into the "male room", but I wonder if that's a defense for the inescapable anxiety of needing to perform on cue in such a strange situation. I remember the first time I had to go into that space for the IUI procedure. Jenna and I had walked into the waiting room and I scribbled my name on the paper fastened to the clipboard. I sat in one of the chairs and pretended to flip through a magazine. When I heard my name called, I looked up to see an attractive woman who greeted me in a friendly tone. She led me down a hallway to a room marked "male room" where she handed me a plastic cup and began rattling off instructions. I don't mind admitting that I was actually fairly nervous, but I tried to make the most of it and laugh off the obvious awkwardness of the moment.

In my mind, I half expected to open the door and find a beautiful hotel room with a huge mahogany bar. I imagined several comfortable couches and chairs to lounge in. A big screen TV with a video playing of Pamela Anderson would monopolize one entire wall, and scantily clad women would serve me filet mignon and iced cold beers while thanking me for my selfless contribution to the cause.

I was quickly brought back to reality as the cold metal door was opened for me. The nurse handed me a few forms to sign. As I handed them back, I started realizing how crazy my life had become. This was not the way I'd dreamed of to conceive our baby.

As soon as the door closed, I got anxious, not knowing how long I was expected to be in there. What if I came out in five minutes? What if I didn't come out for 25 minutes? What were these ladies in the office expecting? It's actually funny to think about this now. At 30 years old, I was staring at a sheet of instructions, worried that I was going to do it wrong! Was there actually a science to this?

One quick survey of the oversized closet I was in proved to me that I was there for a procedure, not the delusion of a vacation. The cracked and worn vinyl recliner brought images to my mind that were not helping my cause. I couldn't get over the idea of how many other guys must have been in this room before me. I totally freaked out. I decided to focus my attention instead to the positives... the porn! But that optimism was shot when I took a cursory glance at the pile of magazines on the table. I'm going to go on a limb that the facility forgot to renew their subscriptions. These magazines were easily over 10 years old. I think even a few of them I saw back when I was in high school. 'Okay, no need to worry,' I thought to myself. 'I still have videos.' But I kid you not when I say that my selection included one, and only one, video of 70's porn! Let's just say there were guys with thick mustaches and women with feathered and frosted hair!

By this time I realized that I had been in there for a while. I wondered what the people on the outside were thinking. I finally settled down on the cold floor with a wrinkled playboy magazine.

While he was away, I sat in the waiting room and flipped through the provided magazines. I don't recall reading a word. Inside my pocket, one hand was fiddling with a rosary that had been given to me from a coworker who swore it was the thing that did the trick for her and her husband. My thumb and forefinger squeeze each segment as I repeated over and over the prayers I had learned in CCD classes.

Mike returned to the waiting room where we sat restlessly until the sperm had been washed to separate the good from the bad. Finally, half an hour later, we were called to an exam room where I waited, legs in stirrups, for our nurse to return. After insertion of the speculum, she took the catheter of sperm and injected them into my cervix. The whole process took just a few minutes and I was stunned at how easy it seemed to be. Lying there for those minutes took weeks, actually years, to be in the making and it was finally over.

In the moments that followed the actual insemination, Mike held my hand as I lay on the table trying to be as still as possible so as not to disrupt the boys in their valiant effort to impregnate me. I had learned that visualization was a reputable method of accomplishing one's goals. So there I was, eyes closed in the sterile room, trying to picture Mike's sperm with little soldier helmets on marching towards a giant egg that was bounding down the fallopian tubes. At one point the boys actually began uttering that "oh-ee-oh-oh-oh" song from the Wizard of Oz. I thought, *that's morbid*, to which they changed their tune to "heigh-ho-heigh-ho it's off to work we go" from Snow White. Much better.

I thought of a lot of other things in that time. I remembered what Mike was wearing when I first met him. I thought about the silly arguments we had over when he was going to finally propose, and I rolled my eyes at how pointless the conversations we had so long ago about Mike not being quite ready to be a father when I first went off birth control pills.

In later minutes, I thought about the future. It was a future I could clearly picture. I had already allowed myself to start feeling hopeful and that hope had brought this moment on the exam table to us. I remember lying there as still as I could and being filled with a sense of optimism and love for the life we had together, and an overwhelming sense of hope for the new life that was certainly coming our way.

All of this was way too serious for Mike, so while I was off fanaticizing a romantic life from the movies, he was looking around the exam room at all of the tools that had been used. His eyes glared at the tools on the metal table. He poked through the cabinets and his eyes contorted when he saw a giant sanitary pad on the counter that I was supposed to use to absorb the excess fluid from the insemination. Ah, yet another experience I would have preferred to keep private.

The Taunting Suppository

Okay, I have eight more days of these disgusting little creamy torpedoes and then I get the verdict to this cycle. If I'm pregnant I will laugh and smile while I insert them, but if not.... I will have humiliated my body in yet another way.

They are the first thing I think about in the morning, even before I have the brain capacity to think at all. At night they have become more essential than my ritual tuck-in and kiss from Mike. On more than one occasion I have found myself dragging my butt out of a warm comfy bed because I forgot the wretched little thing.

I swear they are laughing at me now. Somehow they already know the answer to the crucial question, "Do I need to keep taking these or not?" Sure, they know the answer and they are mocking me each time I put one of those in or each time I wipe the goopy residue off of myself. But maybe they are not mocking me, and instead they are thankful for me taking them as they are feeding the lining where our baby is now growing.

I'm not out of the game. For all I know these irrational thoughts are the hormones of a pregnant woman. After all, in the last 15 minutes I've managed to convince myself they actually have a personality. It's just that right now, this feels like the beginning markers of the downward spiral of insanity. And where will this get me in eight days? Rejection? Rejection for the ... oh I can't even count it out, time, and I won't be able to say that I am stronger for it, or that Mike and I are closer because of this struggle, or that I have seen myself in a new way... no, not a single cliché will make this experience worthwhile. This fluctuation of hope and loss is just a joke of which I seem to be the butt.

I'm trying so hard to stay positive, but I'm incredibly scared. I have let myself become a new person for the sake of this cycle, but the old Jenna keeps scratching her way back. She's not negative; she just wants to protect me from the disappointment. The fact is, no one, not even I, will be able to protect me from that emotion. If this is a bust, there is no way to avoid the disappointment. I might as well just try to enjoy the possibility of a pregnancy for as long as it can last.

The longest two weeks of my life. That's what I was thinking. It's remarkable, really. Prior to infertility, I hadn't really taken note of time as it passed. Sure, there were times when I could feel the clock ticking away; like when I was taking the SAT's in high school, or in the moments before the doors of the church opened and I stood at the end of the aisle looking at Mike on our wedding day.

There we were, staring down 14 days–336 hours– 20,160 minutes. It felt like an eternity. Funny, actually. It had been over two years since I stopped taking birth control pills and started thinking about these children in a serious way. Until this two-week wait, I thought those years had dragged on. But these measly little weeks were far more excruciating. Each day I was painfully aware of how much time I had before the pregnancy test. Mike and I were tempted time and time again to cheat. It seemed like commercials for home pregnancy tests were screaming my name and were playing on a continuous cycle on every channel. I would pick them up, and then put them away. Finally, inevitably, we gave in.

Wednesday, March 30, 2005
And Here I Thought I Was Pretty Smart

So then, why the hell can't I pass this stupid test? Last night Mike and I did a home pregnancy test and it came up negative. I feel stupid, because I was starting to analyze the metallic taste in my mouth and the increasing shortness of breath. I was starting to think the symptoms of the progesterone were really pregnancy symptoms.

I didn't realize how exhausted I was until the test was over. Mike snuggled up behind me on the bed for a while and then after we had some dinner, I fell asleep on the couch. I didn't wake up until hours later and then only to go upstairs and back to sleep. I didn't want to speak or watch TV. I didn't want to think or even dream. I just wanted to be alone and feel the emptiness for a while.

I didn't realize how this would make me feel. How could I feel like I lost something I never had? How is it possible to let go of something I never had my hands on?

This afternoon when I received the call, "I'm sorry I don't have better news," it was more emotionally draining than I had anticipated. I tried to tell Mike that the home test was right and that we needed to prepare for that, but a part of me still had some hope. Mike seemed to have more than a glimmer of hope left. He said things like, "There's still a chance," and when they called and asked me to return their call, I could tell Mike was anxious about why the personal conversation instead of the message on the machine that we usually got. He had called a few times today, but they wouldn't release the information to him without my consent. I have a feeling today was more difficult on him than he anticipated.

I don't know what to do now. Do we take another chuck from our savings? Do we stop this and start to think about adoption while we still have some money left? I've always wanted to adopt, but that was in addition to a biological child, not in substitute for one. But now we are risking both if we don't have money left over. Do we take a break and save more money? I can't believe this didn't work. I can't believe I **didn't work.**

I feel like I disappointed Mike and yes, I know we are a team, but HE did his part. The shots did their part. The

Estrace did its part. The nurse who did the insemination did her part. Who does that leave to blame? What could I have done differently? Was it the wrong meditation CD? Was it the sneezing I did last week? Was it just nerves over the whole thing? Or am I just not meant to be a mother? *NO... absolutely not. I can't even entertain that idea. It's ridiculous and even I don't believe that. We have a lot of options and this was just one small step at the beginning... it's not an end, so stop being dramatic, Jenna.*

Looking at these journal entries now, I have to laugh. The pain was real. The feeling of failure was real, and yet now, when I talk about the number of cycles we've gone through, the first two years and the IUI cycles that followed don't even seem to exist. It's not that they are invalid, or don't deserve the some kind of recognition as the endless cycles of in vitro fertilization (IVF). Truly, they were a difficult time, with a relative amount of worry, disappointment and fear. It is in hindsight that I really am amazed at how far we've come in the journey to parenthood. These early years feel like they belong to someone else; someone far more naïve than the person who writes these words today.

Chapter 4

The Yellow Brick Road Doesn't
Always Lead to the Emerald City

Each step in the infertility process seems like a formidable undertaking. When we went from stopping the pill to taking my temperature, I was amazed that I had even needed to do that. Starting the IUI process was in and of itself, a foreign concept. When we crossed the border to in vitro fertilization (IVF), I was initially intimidated and aghast, unable to recall how we got there. It was like we were caught up in a snowball that became an avalanche of treatment.

If you are experiencing infertility and haven't yet gotten to this stage, I urge you to take this chapter with a grain of salt. Every cycle in the infertility struggle is unique to the individual and is orchestrated by a series of specialists who understand the uniqueness of the patient. I, myself, have never done the same protocol twice in all the years I've been experiencing infertility. Some people experience extreme side effects while others are not affected at all by the hormone fluctuations. Another variable is the length of the cycle. Some women require extra monitoring while others are barely bothered by just a few rounds of blood work or ultrasounds. There are others I have known who become personally invested in every single moment and they have an intense need to know all of the possible outcomes. Others enjoy the "need to know" approach where they simply do what they are told and assume they are in the best hands possible.

But regardless of who you are, how old you are, and what your diagnosis of lack of diagnosis is, a cycle of fertility treatments is often overwhelming and hard to digest for a patient. That is probably the one universal element for all infertile couples. As worrisome and confusing as the processes are to the infertile, I imagine the whole thing must be compounded for the fertiles in their life.

As a fertile you may feel uncomfortable asking your loved one what they are doing and how much they are taking in terms of medication. This is, after all, private information. The point of this next section is to illustrate one example of a fresh IVF cycle. It may not mirror exactly, but it will provide you with a sense of how incredibly time consuming, as well as how emotionally and financially draining, this process is. If you don't feel comfortable asking the down and dirty questions of your loved one, but still very much want to empathize with their struggle, perhaps this section with be of help.

It's important to note that many infertiles who begin treatments never need to undergo more invasive procedures than those described in my IUI journal segments. In fact, according to The American Society for Reproductive Medicine, only 3% of infertility patients will require any kind of advanced reproductive assistance. This means that if you have a loved one who is experiencing IVF and they tell you they feel alone, you ought to believe them. They aren't being dramatic. I was the first person in my circle of friends to have difficulty conceiving. While the others around me were getting pregnant in the first few months of trying, I felt alone, depressed, confused, and I didn't think there was anywhere to turn. It wasn't that I couldn't confide in my fertile friends, but their worlds were revolving around nurseries and baby showers. We just weren't in the same places in our lives. I didn't share my experiences with anyone for the first two years because I thought I was broken, physically and mentally. Thank goodness for the internet and its message boards. The women there became my friends, pseudo-therapists and shoulders to cry on. They understood the struggles of infertility first hand and knew when a pep talk was in order and when to simply empathize.

After our second failed IUI, it was clear that we needed to consider other options. We had already spent half of our savings on the treatments, testing, and other procedures to determine what might be the actual issue behind my infertility. If it was simply that I didn't ovulate, the process afforded by artificial insemination should have rectified that. After all, I was ovulating, and even ovulating multiple eggs. Mike's sperm should have been getting women pregnant who walked by him. So what was it? I thought we had already pulled out the big guns.

When we heard the term "in vitro fertilization," images of latex gloved, surgical-masked doctors and nurses mixing magic potions in a sterile room came to mind. I had done my homework on IUI, but this was the big daddy of infertility treatments. On the message boards I had visited, these women had their own little neighborhoods where the amateurs like me just could not enter. I had heard of "test tube" babies and like most civilians, I thought this was just the way infertile women got pregnant. I remember thinking, *How much easier could it be? All I have to do is lay there while they place the baby inside of me. Even I can handle that!*

But there were still decisions to make. We had to consider the financial aspect first. It had taken us eight years to get where we were. We were young, but ahead of the game. We had a dog, two cats, two cars, and a beautiful home in an upper middle-class neighborhood. Mike, being the financial guy, had started us on retirement plans through our first employment situations out of college. Now, slowly, aspects of that life were being compromised for a marginal chance at parenthood.

This is probably a good time to interject the story with the explanation of the guilt factor. As we talked with the people closest to us, looking for some objective feedback, we would hear things like, "I would sell my house if I had to," or "There's nothing I wouldn't give and no price that I wouldn't pay for my child." So how could we not try? It felt like the obvious answer. How materialistic were we being to even suggest that there wasn't money for the necessary procedures?

This is not to suggest that Mike and I wouldn't have come to this decision on our own. I'm certain that in speaking to friends, we were subconsciously looking for a reason to bite the bullet and write the check. It's just that with their words came a feeling of selfishness that made the decision to spend the remainder of our savings, in addition to a contribution from my parents easier to digest.

If there was any question in our minds about rolling the financial dice on IVF instead of putting it into something like adoption, we felt convinced after speaking to our doctor. Our specialist explained that they were seeing recent successes that were near 60% in the last month or two for women in my age range. This was three times the success rate that we were up against with the IUI. Furthermore, over three rounds, our chances of conceiving were near 90%. For the first time we were on the BETTER side of the odds. It was going to cost us around $11,000, but we had to compare this to the significantly higher price of adoption. In addition, there was the real possibility that we could be pregnant in two months instead of the year or more estimated wait for adoption; the path to a family seemed entirely clear.

A word from Mike:

I couldn't believe how expensive an IVF procedure was. There was a stretch of about two months where a day wouldn't go by without receiving a medical bill in the mail. It didn't take long for the savings to deplete entirely. We were fortunate to have Jenna's parents generously helping us with some of the payments, but we were adults who were bringing in very good salaries. Call it pride or a need to be self-sufficient, but I didn't want to rely on my in-laws for money as if I was a teenager depending on an allowance.

We eventually had to do a credit card advance for the procedure. It made me cringe as I called the credit card company for the money. What could I do? It's extremely difficult for me not to get angry when I talk about this topic. My financial goals were put on hold indefinitely. My excel spreadsheet was showing zeros in the additional principle column. I was paying interest on credit card balances because I couldn't afford to pay them off.

Fear starting to set in on how many cycles we could afford to do IVF. We talked about the possibility of selling our house and downsizing our cars to free up additional

---

cash each month. We felt guilty when we ordered out and became increasing more aware of unnecessary lights that were on in the house. We had to save all our money to combat the infertility demon. I was also getting depressed because I knew once we had children, it would be a long road just to pay off the current debt. Plans of Jenna taking time off to care for the baby were distant memories.

I started to become jealous of my married friends. They were all taking their non-infertility money and putting it towards other things, like house improvements, dining room sets, and increasing their retirement contributions. Jenna and I kept taking steps backwards.

Part One: Suppression:

It started with a cycle of birth control pills. Yep, that's right. The nemesis of the infertile is actually part of the process towards conception. But it isn't as simple as it was in my teenage years, when popping a pill once a day was done without thought. It was the beginning of the game. It would be five weeks before a baby was even possible and almost two months before we would come to the day when we would know if the injections and monitoring, praying and faith, had resulted in success. In the time that a fertile will have two chances to get pregnant, the IVF patient will pin their hopes, and often their bank account, on just one chance.

Three weeks of birth control will test the patience of even the strongest infertile. For three weeks it felt like we were going backwards, further and further from the dream. There was no hope for a miracle baby during those three weeks. I didn't ovulate without the pill, I certainly wasn't about to start ovulating while on it. We were actually taking conscious efforts with each pill to prevent the very thing we wanted so badly. Sure, there was the occasional story of the girl who got pregnant while on the pill, and there was always the dismal hope that maybe that would happen. This, however, was too remote to be more than a punch line.

To say this was a bitter pill to swallow was an understatement. In the good old days, these pills meant freedom to have sex without a fear of pregnancy. How ironic it was that with each pill I took during the suppression stage of IVF, the less I wanted to engage in that kind of experience. *What's the point? Oh yeah, this is supposed to be fun, right?* How times had changed! By that point, I had been poked and prodded by more people than I could have ever imagined. It was hard to remember a time when my reproductive organs were used for anything beyond scientific experimentation.

Part Two: The Stimulation Phase

After weeks of pill popping each day, I began the first of many injections. I was still a few days away from stopping the birth control altogether, so there was a bit of overlap in the medication. That first injection marked the last time I would be able to breathe easy for a long time. From this point forward, I needed to prepare and deliver my own injections and my daily routines needed to revolve around a series of appointments for monitoring. Each morning, it was the first thing I thought about when I woke up. It had to be. If I forgot my perfectly timed injection, I knew I was risking ovulation at an inopportune time, which could send the cycle, literally, into the toilet. So at 6:45 each morning, just as I was about to head to work, I first kissed Mike good-bye and then went to the bathroom to get my shot ready. I sat on the toilet and amassed a bit of fat around my belly button where I injected the medication called Lupron, a medication that would prevent me from ovulating before I was ready. Then, off I went to school to live life with a secret hope in my heart.

Wednesday, May 25, 2005

Lupron Day 1... The Beginning

This morning I gave myself the first of many Lupron shots. I've been anticipating this day for more than a month now and finally we are getting started. Technically, we started the cycle with the first birth control pill, but that just seemed like a waste of time to me. I've been counting down the days to get to the real stuff and now we are finally here. I'm having some anxiety about this whole thing and I'm not sure if it's due to the anticipation of possibly being pregnant, or if it's from the nervousness of having it turn out negative.

This morning as I was giving myself that first shot, I realized the gravity of the situation. This wasn't like the IUI injections when slowly my body would start to produce a relatively normal amount of follicles and in theory, I could conceive our baby in my own body. This was the first of many shots that will produce a completely unnatural response in my body. And once I have grown dozens of follicles, they will be surgically removed from me and somewhere in an unknown laboratory our babies will be conceived. I sat on the toilet holding the first Lupron shot and I came to the sudden realization that I won't even be present when our babies begin their journey to life. Logically, I suppose I already knew this, but in that moment when the theory of IVF became a reality, it was hard to truly comprehend.

I feel sick about this. I wonder if we made the right decision.

We want to be parents. There is no easy answer to how to make this happen. I've been told to "relax" and that I can't force this to work. Still, literally everything we have is riding on this. How is it realistic to not feel stress over this? I suppose being told to relax is the only thing some people can come up with. If they haven't put their financial and emotion future on the line for something, relaxing must seem like a very reasonable response.

This could be the beginning of the rest of my life, or it could be the beginning of the end. We are heading towards a reality that is incomprehensible... either way. After all this time I can't imagine it not turning out for the best, and yet as I read the stories of women who have gone through this, I am finding women on their second, third and fourth tries without success. How would we be able to do that?

I can't do anything that I will later regret. I can't afford any "if only I had..." moments. What am I missing? What have I forgotten? What will I be kicking myself for later?

A few days went by of this routine, one injection each morning, and due to the end of the birth control, I got my period. Finally, a predictable period! This is the one and only time that a period was not only welcomed, but praised. It meant a fresh start. A clean slate, so to speak, and the beginning of possibility. Unfortunately, I would be remiss if I failed to mention that it was also the beginning of a long journey that is not for the faint at heart, or those with an intense need for privacy. Over the next several weeks my body will become much like a NASCAR vehicle. Like the finely skilled professionals at the racetrack, there will be countless people observing, poking, and reviewing every aspect of my body. They will use instruments that make strange noises, and measure parts of me that aren't viewable to the naked eye. Check your ego and humility at the door, and get ready to board the roller coaster that is the

IVF stimulation cycle.

First things first; welcome to the laboratory. With close to $4,500 worth of medication, including four different types and sizes of needles, two weeks' worth of two different vaginal suppositories, and two oral medications, I was stunned by the notion that all of the little vials and packages contained medication that in cost rivaled two mortgage payments! Literally, that was tough to swallow. Mike and I began to organize yet another part of our lives around infertility. This time the disease even had its own room. Tucked away during the day, or when company was over, the pharmacy covered the entire counter space of the master bathroom. It became such a disruption in our otherwise normal lives that we made the decision to keep the door closed when it wasn't in use, just to get a reprieve from it.

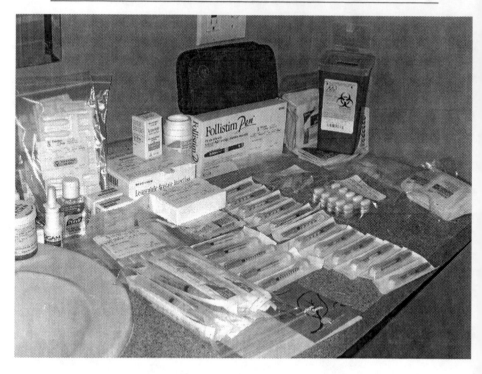

Bathroom pharmacy ready for customers

But that wouldn't be nearly as easy as shutting the door. Some of the medications required refrigeration, so as best as we could, we tucked away the yet to be used drugs into a drawer between the fresh fruits and the deli meats. We wrapped the boxes in grocery bags so that they wouldn't create unnecessary questions when people fetched a cold soda or a snack.

With our first IVF, we felt like we were living a double life. Each weekday we were going to work like normal functioning people. We came home, ate dinner, watched television, and talked about our days. But at night our schedule was completely dictated by the timing of the shots. When it was time to do an injection, we were all business, getting the job done and trying not to think, and over think, the possibilities of what each injection could be doing deep inside of me.

And that double life existed within my own personality as well. On a dime I could change my outlook on an entire cycle based on one blood draw or a single ultrasound. Sometimes I found myself optimistic and even grateful for the opportunity to experience such a miracle of science. I was fascinated by the entire process and in admiration of the women who had gone through it half a dozen times. then, just like snapping my fingers, suddenly I felt myself falling into a pit of self-pity, angry that I was alone in my experiences and scared of the possibility that I might end up like one of those sad cases; trying for years and years with nothing to show for it but an endless stack of medical bills and eternal guilt over the failures. And the craziest part was that these emotions were the natural ones. The side effects from the hormonal medications hadn't even begun to take their toll.

Monday, May 30, 2005

Hopeaholic vs. The Pessimiser

Okay, so who is this crazy person who is overcome by fifteen different emotions? Well, Hopeaholic (hence forward deemed "Hope") feels like these are the multiple emotions of a pregnant woman whose hormones are just off the wall. Every day, Hope holds onto the cross that her friend gave her. She rubbed it on her tummy during the IUIs and while Mike was engaged in his donations to the cause. Hope looks at the stats and is confident that there is no reason why I can't be one of those for whom this type of procedure will work. She even smiles at the idea that twins might result. It was her idea to religiously use the meditation CD each evening and she's excited about the possibility of having acupuncture.

The Pessimiser (hence forth deemed "Pissy") is a much different personality. Pissy is controlling, confident and well established here. I dare to think she has been around the longest. She will stand astute with her glasses on and explain very matter-of -factly that the percentage of women who find success in the IVF process is still only around 50% regardless of what the last couple of months had generated for this particular clinic. Pissy looks at the CDC website and realizes that other clinics have better stats and questions whether the best possible choice was made. The only reasonable conclusion Pissy can come to is that any excitement would be premature and simply unfounded.

It's a good thing both of these personalities are among the group gathered compactly in my body. Without them, I am certain I would have been pushed over the edge years ago. But as I approach the final days before the IVF stimulation cycle can begin, I admit that Hope is most welcome to dominate the conversations. She's shy though, so who knows if she will show her face much. When this cycle is over, it will be Pissy that will anxiously host the Pity Party with her theme song "I Told You So" blaring through the room. But Hope will arrive with a platter of "Don't Ever Give Up" and a cooler filled with "You're Stronger than You Realize". She always brings the best comfort foods.

And so it began. Cycle day two meant the baseline of everything. This is the most important first impression for the infertile. Blood work would indicate where my hormones were starting at and the ultrasound gives us the first look at the sleeping ovaries that are hiding the possibility of life. If the impression is right, the cycle can proceed and there will be every reason to feel optimistic about our future. It sounds like an amazing moment of unrealized potential. The reality is it's not that romantic. The day two ultrasound is done on exactly that; the second day of the cycle. That means that as I lay on the exam table with my legs firmly in stirrups, I was not really thinking about the beauty of life beginning. I was thinking, *Please don't let this be a bloody mess on the ultrasound lady!"* When the wand was inserted, I was praying for the moment to be over with the least humiliation possible. It had slid in easily and I knew it wasn't from any synthetic lubrication. *Oh my God, don't look.* Sure, the ultrasonographer is probably used to it. This is just part of her job. But it isn't part of mine. She was a great sport about the whole thing and talked lightheartedly as she moved it around and took measurements. And then it was withdrawn. *Ughhh.* I jumped from the table and used the stack of paper towels to wipe myself up. The woman didn't even have time to leave the room before I was dressed and ready to go. This is just one of the many experiences that many fertile people do not consider when they think of infertility treatments. Infertility isn't pretty. It invades the most private aspects of life and demands humility at each step.

Day two is also the day when the medications kick into full gear. In my case, it began with a massive dose of an antibiotic for both Mike and I in order to stave off any infections. When I first heard of this, it seemed like no big deal. In comparison to the needles and suppositories that were lined up on my bathroom counter, one big horse pill was child's play. WRONG! An hour and a half after taking the pill, Mike and I realized how truly important it was to have two bathrooms in our home. For the next four hours we didn't see each other for more than fifteen minutes. Apparently the warning of "may cause stomach upset" was a major underestimation of the fact. If it wasn't coming out one end, it was coming out the other. My head was spinning and cold sweat was flooding out of every pore. Between the ultrasound and the antibiotic, I knew this IVF business was going to be a hard uphill haul.

A word from Mike:

I must admit, I was relieved when Jenna was able to give herself the shots in her stomach. I've never been especially comfortable sticking a sharp pointed object into anything. The idea of a pin popping a balloon is enough to make me shudder. So when Jenna began the injections, I helped with getting things ready, but when it came time to actually stick the needle in her stomach, I turned away. Nonetheless, after watching her a few nights the idea sort of intrigued me. I wanted to see how much it hurt getting a shot in the stomach. It was just a ½ inch needle. My stomach had a decent amount of cushion as well that had built up over the past few years. I almost jumped as Jenna put the needle in my stomach. No thanks! I don't see how I could do that every day.

I spent the next two weeks preparing two injections each morning and another at night. In addition, I was continuing to use the vaginal suppository of Estrace to thicken up my stubborn endometrial lining. Every other morning, I woke up an extra half hour early to get to the clinic for monitoring. Either it was a blood draw or an ultrasound, or both. Sitting in the waiting room caused a myriad of emotions to bubble to the surface. The women around me had the same expressions. It was like waiting for a surprise party or an execution. No one knew which fate was to be theirs. The tension was palpable. At any time, I knew the results of these tests could make or break my cycle.

What's worse than sitting quietly in a waiting room

with a bunch of other infertiles whose hormones are also skyrocketing and worried about the same tests? That's easy. It's baby day! Once a week at my clinic, all of the women who have found success in the month or weeks before come in for the one day a week when my doctor holds ultrasounds. It is inevitable I would hit this day at least once a cycle. Their expression is different. They avoid eye contact with the infertiles. Perhaps it's a sense of guilt or empathy for having what we want, or maybe it's a fear that if they look at us they will be turned back into infertile stone like the ancient story of Medusa. Whatever it is, time never passed more slowly than on the days when I was surrounded by happy couples thumbing through magazines and whispering about their new found happiness.

Wednesday, June 1, 2005

Losers to the Left

I walked into the clinic for what has become a very predictable part of my daily routine, like brushing my teeth and walking the dog. But unlike those other things, being there always gives me a mixed sense of emotions. I am anxious to see how things are progressing, but worried no matter what I learn. Is it good news, is it bad? Today was definitely bad, but not because of the results of any testing. When I walked in the door, I found myself in the middle of Baby Day. I might as well have walked into the pit of hell. There were five couples who were awaiting their ultrasound after becoming pregnant. The snuggled up close to each other and I could just feel their sense of excitement permeate the still air of the office. Some of them were smiling ear to ear, but I was grateful that they tried to keep their enthusiasm to a minimum. That came to an abrupt halt when another woman walked in the door with what appeared to be her entire extended family. They were laughing and giddy, and entirely inappropriate. It was something I would have expected in an OB/GYN office where the pregnant ladies don't know anything about the infertile world. But this woman! Obviously she'd had some kind of struggle and she should have known better than to gallivant into that office like that. It was purely insensitive.

And worse than this was that I had to sit and wait for each person to go in and come out before it was my turn. It wasn't that I got there last. No, apparently on Baby Day, the doctor has to see all the pregnant ultrasounds before he can go to surgery at the hospital, so they allow all the pregnant women to usurp the regular infertiles in line. So I sat there. And I sat there. I watched three couples come out and proudly show their ultrasounds to the nurses, and one couple come out screaming with joy at twins. I could feel their happiness squeeze my heart. I haven't felt so empty in a long time. A final couple left quietly after learning that there was no developing fetus. I'm not sure which of these was harder to take as I sat there in a puddle of self-pity.

It was a miserable experience and I so badly wanted to not be there. When the nurse was drawing my blood, it was all I could do to not cry. She looked at me and I explained in my best non-confrontational way that it was incredibly uncomfortable to sit there with those women and that maybe they should consider having these women in later in the morning or on a separate day. I tried to jokingly suggest that they should have a "losers' lounge" where the rest of the infertiles could toss back shots of espresso. I would have gladly gone there.

The nurse responded that I should feel hope at seeing this, not jealous. No one gets it. Not even the people who do this for a living. I am not jealous of these women. They deserve to have their babies. I don't think I have earned that role more or less than any of them. This isn't a competition. Their happiness doesn't make me jealous; it just makes me sad for myself.

My clinic has quoted statistics to me since the day we walked in for our first consultation. Their stats are supposed to make me feel comforted and excited. I must refer here to Newton's Law of Motion: for every action there is an equal and opposite reaction. In this particular case, for every pregnant woman in that office, there has to be a non pregnant woman. That's me today. It's been me every day since 2003.

In between all of the shots and appointments for monitoring, life goes on. Despite the stereotype of the desperate people who cry every night over not being able to have a baby, infertile people do actually function in normal society. One of the most insulting pieces of advice that I was ever given in my years of struggling with this disease was when a person quoted to me, "Life is what happens when you're busy making other plans." In other words, I was spending my life futilely trying to have children and in the meantime, the good things in my world were passing me by. That person could not have been more wrong.

Infertility had made me more grateful and more aware of what Mike and I had built for ourselves. With the commotion of infertility running around in my head and heart, I looked for solace in every ordinary place. Whether it was making a dinner of Mike's favorite foods, landscaping our yard over the summers, or working on my first young adolescent novel, my life moved forward, and so did I.

If I was spending every moment consumed with infertility, I would not have been able to function for my 90 seventh graders on a daily basis. As I raced to school after a blood draw that would inevitably make me late for homeroom, I pulled myself together. On a day where good news ran abundant, I tucked away the excitement and focused on the writing project that my students were working on. On a bad day, I still raced to school, but I wiped away the tears and forced myself to think about the next eight hours of work ahead of me. Either way, when I walked into my classroom, those students got the very best of me that I had to offer. I contributed to the success of their education every day, and I would like to think that even on my worst days, I didn't miss an opportunity to crack a corny joke or make a connection between our lessons and their real lives. In some ways it was those children, the people who knew nothing of our struggle, who gave me the greatest relief from the rollercoaster of daily emotions. They were compassionate without even realizing it, and on the days that I was having a tough time keeping it all together, they seemed to sense it and metamorphosed on cue to adjust to what was needed.

I didn't wish away my life or spend my nights wallowing in the "why me?" of infertility. Of course those moments came and sometimes they were frequent and stayed around a little longer than I would have desired. I admit I would often want to speed through a day to see what message was on the machine when I got home so that I'd know the results from the morning's blood draw. But as often as I spent time dealing with this disease, there were the moments of having a beer after work with girlfriends, or camping out on the couch and watching a movie with my husband, or babysitting our nephew. And, although infertility may have been on my mind, so was the Christmas shopping we had to do and the toilet I hadn't cleaned in a week. Infertility was a part of our life, but it wasn't our entire life.

Certainly the monitoring and stimulation phase of an IVF cycle is a massive effort on the part of the patients and the doctors. Because of this, there were times when we did have to plan certain aspects of our life around injections and such. If there was a dinner party at a friend's house, we had to be sure that we could get home in time for the 8 p.m. injection. Other times we had to decline a weekend getaway because I had to be at the clinic early in the morning for an ultrasound. And there were even times when we would be traveling and Mike would have to pull into a fast food restaurant so that I could go into the bathroom and take care of business.

Saturday, June 4, 2005

Shooting Up in the McDonald's

Last night Mike and I found ourselves in another interesting predicament. We had been out visiting family and we knew we probably weren't going to make it home in time for the shots, so we decided to take them with us. The plan was that I would excuse myself to the bathroom and do the injection some point around our normal medication time. The problem was, both of us forgot. We were having such a great time that we lost track of time and for once, we actually lost track of this cycle.

On the way home, I went into a panic. I was afraid I would miss the window of opportunity where the injection needed to be taken. I could just picture going for monitoring tomorrow and having them tell me that I had missed a dose and we would need to cancel the whole thing. Logically, I suppose I knew that wasn't going to be the case, but we had been so good about remembering every medication, I just didn't want this to be the one time we messed up. Mike didn't think that being off by an hour or two was going to make much of a difference, but I just couldn't get it out of my head. He kept saying, "What's the worst case scenario?" Obviously that would be a cancelled cycle and dropping another couple thousand to start over... I won that argument!

We pulled into a McDonald's and I took my baggie of supplies

59

to the bathroom. It was absolutely filthy in there, so I sat on the toilet and tried to build a little space on my lap where I could prepare everything. I had the medication measured out and had just finished cleaning the spot to inject when a woman walked into the bathroom. I looked up at the door to my stall and noticed that in my haste I had forgotten to lock it! There was no way I could get up. My lap was covered in supplies and I had the needle cap dangling out of my mouth. I prayed that she would knock or see my feet if she looked under, but before I could do anything, she had pushed open the door. Oh my God... the embarrassment! For both of us! She glared at me and I could see her fix her eyes on the vial on my lap and the needle hanging out of my stomach. There was nothing I could do. She shut the door and raced out of the bathroom. She didn't even try to go into another stall.... What must she have been thinking?

Obviously she was thinking I was doing drugs in the bathroom stall of McDonald's... and she was right.

By the beginning of the second week of medications and monitoring, the real side effects of the drugs began to kick in. Certainly every patient responds differently to the hormonal drugs, but I think it's important to spend some time on this, because if you are the loved one of an infertility patient this might be a very difficult aspect of the cycle to grasp. For me, this one week before the eggs were ready to be retrieved were physically painful and emotionally exhausting.

I have always been very sensitive to medication. Whether it's cold medicine or inhalers for asthma, I have usually been prescribed the lowest dose or the child's version. Even non-drowsy medications would leave my head spinning. With IVF, there was no child's dose, which meant I was on my own to deal with the fallout. Every side effect from all medications, I had the displeasure of experiencing, often simultaneously.

The doses of the medications involved in stimulating the ovaries to produce multiple follicles will invariably produce hormone levels that can feel out of control. Migraine headaches, dizziness, loss of concentration, and fatigue were the more pleasant aspects of my treatment. At the same time, I was often constipated, bloated, and completely irrational in my emotions. I'm fairly certain that Mike is the most patient man I know because looking back on these cycles now, I can see why anyone would want to run from the room when I walked in.

I often gave my very best to the kids at school, which meant that in the weeks where the drugs were circulating, I was running on empty when I dragged myself into the house. The lights were usually off when he came home from work, but not because I was sleeping. I would be parked on the couch with a throbbing headache and unable to handle any lights or noises. No amount of aspirin would bring me comfort.

When I started the cycle I weighed about 104 pounds. In the days before the egg retrieval procedure, I would usually be at around 115. In just a few weeks I would not only feel the exhaustion of the extra pounds, but I couldn't wear my own clothes. The bloating in my abdomen required me to purchase a few special pairs of pants or reduce my active wardrobe to certain looser skirts and dresses. Even my clothing was compromised by the cycle.

It was a truly miserable week or so leading up to the retrieval, but honestly, every shot was a blessing to us. Each time we had a blood draw or ultrasound, we knew we were getting closer to the day when I would be pregnant. With each injection that burned or left me nauseous, I was concentrating on the distinct possibility of that shot being the one shot to help create the follicle that would contain the egg that would be fertilized, that would be transferred and may implant to eventually grow into our baby. It was like the Mother Goose rhyme, "This is the House that Jack Built". But this was the baby that IVF built. At the end of the rhyme we'd forget how it started, but it would all be well worth the trouble it took to get there.

Part Three: The Egg Retrieval

Ten days after that nightmarish first ultrasound, the day arrived for which we had hoped. No, we weren't pregnant. For IVF patients, every positive step, even a small one, is worth celebrating. We received the phone call explaining that it was time for the "trigger shot". This one shot is possibly the most important injection of the entire cycle. It is critical that it is delivered at a very precise time according to the instructions of the clinic. The trigger shot is basically a massive dose of Human Chorionic Gonadotropin (hCG). In pregnant women, it is the hormone produced by the human placenta. It's the same hormone that makes the pretty little + sign on the home pregnancy tests. In an IVF patient, it is used to trigger ovulation. It stimulates the eggs to mature and be released from the ovary. In exactly 36 hours from administering this shot, the eggs will be extracted through a surgical procedure called the "egg retrieval." This is a truly exciting time. Other than the fact that the aftermath of this shot felt much like a tetanus shot, lingering for a few days, the whole cycle seemed to be refueled with the adrenaline of hope.

Thursday, June 9, 2005
So Close and Hanging on

Today's blood work came back and the results are in. We are triggering tonight and are planning on the retrieval for Saturday morning.

I'm so nervous right now. I feel like I can start to get excited, and yet, I'm so nervous to think about it actually happening. I have one more blood work up and I know too well how important that is. Anything can happen. They could decide to retrieve the eggs and fertilize them, but not proceed with the transfer if the hormones levels are too high or they fear hyperstimulation. If the numbers go down they could think we aren't responding as well as we should, and perhaps the egg quality will be compromised..

Anxiety... this is a big part of my life right now. I have so many questions that there are no answers for through my usual research methods. How many eggs will we get? How many will fertilize? Will they cancel my transfer? And of course, ultimately, will it succeed and we'll be pregnant? Only time or a psychic friend holds these answers.

It's time to get back to the optimism I used to have each month. This IVF has really thrown me for a loop. I was mentally prepared for how time-consuming the shots and the monitoring would be, but I hadn't anticipated the physical effects of the medications at these levels or the drain this would take on my emotional state. Sometimes I think my need to understand the process has been my greatest strength, and at the same time, my worst enemy. I have a too proficient level of comprehension about each step in the process, hormone level and side effect. While that has helped us to make some important decisions about our treatment and be proactive on this course, I realize there is something to be said for kicking back and just doing what I'm told. I promised myself never to be misguided by doctors who claim to be experts, but I know I'm certainly no physician myself. Where's the middle ground of naïveté and neurosis?

I need to allow myself to accept that there really is nothing more that I can do and that the rest is up to God and the doctors. It's so hard to let go of the control and allow the vulnerability of the situation to enter my mind. But the fact is, I've been vulnerable now for years. I've never *really* had control over any of this, and when I tried to take control, I ended up with the defeat and guilt of a failed cycle.

Things moved quickly in the 36 hours following the shot. While we waited for the retrieval hour to approach, the house was a bustle with cleaning and cooking. I was busy preparing meals for the four days of bed rest that were impending. Mike was cleaning the whole house from top to bottom. Laundry was done, folded and put away. Toilets were cleaned and every piece of furniture was vacuumed. Empty microwavable containers were lined up on the kitchen counter awaiting a variety of lunches and dinners to be frozen and stored away. In a strange way, it was a nesting period where we were preparing for the arrival of our embryos.

The morning of the egg retrieval I woke up early. I grabbed a quick shower, but didn't use any shampoo or soap. I had heard that any kind of fragrance could affect the eggs and whether that was or wasn't true, I knew that I didn't want to take any chances. I was aware of a dozen reasons why a retrieval could have been cancelled at any point during our cycle, so I knew I was fortunate to get that far.

I hadn't eaten anything since dinner the previous night and thankfully, I wasn't hungry. I wasn't allowed to eat because the procedure at the hospital would have me under general anesthesia. Nervousness and excitement was keeping my stomach full enough. Of course this wasn't the only thing that had reserved a place inside of me. The trigger shot had enlarged the size of the eggs in order to give them one final push towards maturity. If you can imagine carrying a tennis ball filled with sand under the skin on either side of your belly button you might be able to grasp the kind of discomfort I'm talking about here. The weight and pressure from my ovaries and the follicles that had grown was nearly unbearable. It had even become slightly difficult to breathe in the last 24 hours. My most comfortable running pants were too tight. I changed into a pair of pajama bottoms and a baggy sweatshirt, and we were off to the hospital.

I was surprised how efficient everything was when we got there. Mike and I were taken into a private room where the nurses were all incredibly happy. I realized this must be a fantastic area to work in. Everyone who comes in must be full of excitement or trepidation, but regardless of which, there was always possibility. Like an assembly line in a manufacturing plant, nurses came through time and time again. One drew blood, another inserted the IV, and others asked questions. I remember thinking how funny it was when one nurse came in, looked up from her clipboard, and smiled. "I have to ask this. Is there any chance you could be pregnant?" I laughed out loud at the absurdity of the question, which only made my ovaries feel more uncomfortable. It was a great ice breaker.

Finally the anesthesiologist came in. Mike kissed me on the forehead and I was guided into the operating room with my butt half hanging out of the jonnie. Once on the table, it was all work for the staff and all fun for me. Heart monitors were stuck to my chest and people I had never met before came into the room wearing gowns that made it difficult to determine even their gender. With an oxygen mask covering my mouth, I began the most peaceful sleep of my life.

Up until the moment I was put under, I didn't think there could be a more uncomfortable aspect to the IVF cycle than the days prior to the retrieval. With the weight gain from ovarian stimulation and the medication side effects, I was ready, willing and able to do whatever it took to get those eggs out of me. If I had to walk on my hands to get to the hospital, I would have gladly done so. I was anticipating a literal sigh of relief once they were gone. I was so wrong.

Upon waking up in the recovery room, I genuinely thought someone was sitting on me. The pressure on my abdomen was unreal. Every inch of me was trembling from the aftermath of the anesthesia and I was freezing cold in the core of my body. The kind nurses returned to wrap me in several warm blankets until only my eyes, nose and mouth were exposed to my surroundings. In the groggy state of semi-consciousness, I began asking the question that would be repeated at least ten times before I would recall having already asked it. "How many did they get?"

Within a half hour several specialists visited us. The first was our RE. He explained to us that they extracted 18 eggs. We were overjoyed. In our minds, eighteen eggs meant the equivalent of 18 months of trying by a normal fertile person. It was like someone had just dropped the biggest present in our laps. The news continued to pour in. The andrologist who was in charge of looking over Mike's contribution, said his numbers were fantastic and far better than any of his past sperm samples. Lastly, an embryologist visited with us to let us know that she would call the next day to let us know how many were fertilized, but that we had every reason to expect great news on that end.

Part Four: The Embryo Transfer

The day after the retrieval was hell for a number of reasons. I hadn't been able to move effectively since I did the trigger shot and as much as thought I would feel relief from having the eggs removed, I was sorely mistaken, literally. As long as I was lying down on my back, gravity was my friend. All of the aches could sink into the couch and I watched television happily comforted by my newest friend, the painkiller Percocet. As soon as I moved to the side, it was like a sandbag inside of my abdomen would roll onto any innocent organ and threaten to crush it. Forget standing. The few times I got up to use the bathroom, I thought for sure all of my organs that hadn't been crushed were going to fall out of my vagina. What I initially thought was a two-hundred pound man sitting *on* my stomach, suddenly felt more like a two-hundred pound man sitting *inside* my stomach. It was a restless night after the retrieval. Not only was I physically uncomfortable, but Mike and I were also naturally worried about how the eggs and sperm were doing. In theory they should have been uniting, but we knew better than to make assumptions or take anything for granted.

One day post retrieval, another moment of high anxiety set in. Just because they retrieved a number of eggs did not guarantee that any of those would actually fertilize. They could have been immature or of poor quality. I was well aware of the possibility that any number of obstacles would still need to be overcome before we made it to the time when any embryos might be transferred back to me. When I called the clinic the morning after the retrieval, I was holding my breath as I had done so many times during the cycle.

Sunday, June 12, 2005
AHHHHHH

I don't think I slept more than two hours last night. And even when I did sleep, I was dreaming about today. I didn't want to get too excited, but I just had a feeling it was going to be great news. This morning, the first thing we did after waking up was to call the clinic to find out the news. Of course they didn't have the fertilization report ready, but at least I got to leave a message so they would know that I was going to keep calling until there was an answer. Then around 11 a.m. the call came in.

Remarkably, 16, yes **16 of the 18 fertilized!!!!** They want me to call back tomorrow to find out when they will do the transfer. Right now they are thinking it might not be until Thursday. As much as I'd love to have them back as soon as possible, I know letting them grow a bit more will allow them to weed out the less competent ones and only keep the others.

I'm ecstatic that this is all starting to happen. It's a relief to know that my eggs aren't a total disaster and that we should have some that will work for the transfer. I know that most of the ones that fertilized probably won't make it and even if they do, we still need them to implant.

But that's another day, and so for today I need to concentrate on keeping the possibility of hyper-stimulation at bay. I weighed in at 114 pounds just before the operation and if I gain more than five pounds they will cancel the transfer. I've been plying myself with water and trying to relax. I could probably go back to work tomorrow, but I'm taking the day off to relax more and try to get my body ready for the big days ahead. Funny how suddenly I couldn't care less about how many sick days I have or what the kids at school are going to do without me. I may have some of my own children to worry about soon! Yikes! I can't believe I just wrote that!

Can I say, AHHHHHHHHHHHHHHHH

68

Mike and I were on cloud nine. If there was a cloud 15 we would have happily skipped over to that one, too. Excitement glowed in every room of the house. We were reenergized, not just by the news of the fertilized eggs, but we felt proud of ourselves for facing the infertility obstacle and coming out on the other side. The elation of the cycle transformed even the pain of the retrieval to a simple nuisance.

In the next few days I took care of all of the school work that needed to be done. I didn't want to be worried about taking care of my students when I really needed to take care of myself. It was good to return to work for a few days to give my mind a reprieve from IVF for a while. I had lost a bit of the balance I was maintaining in the excitement of the past few days.

Finally, a few days after the retrieval, we were scheduled to return to the hospital for the transfer of our embryos. An hour before the procedure, I swallowed the required dose of valium which would relax the uterus and accept the embryos. I also began tackling the 32 ounces of water that was needed to make the transfer easier to maneuver.

There are only a few times during my IVF experience where I can say it was actually "fun". This was one of those. As miserably as I was handling the side effects of the hormonal medications, the bright side was that I was equally sensitive to the valium. It was really having an effect on my ability to form a coherent sentence. When our RE came into the room to give us paperwork to sign, I busted out in a laughter that actually brought me to tears. It was one of the few times I had laughed during the cycle and the release was something I desperately needed. Unfortunately, it may have been slightly inappropriate, because my signature couldn't be accepted on the release form, so Mike had to cosign in order to proceed. The nurses were laughing and joking with Mike about how I was a "cheap date" and that this was the most fun a transfer had been in a while.

With my feet placed in the stirrups once again, and my bottom half fully exposed to the infantry of specialists who entered the room, I was in a very familiar position. I warned the doctor that my bladder felt so full that I was worried about peeing on him, but he insisted that had only happened once. The idea of this led me to laugh even more hysterically. Everyone in the room had to pause their parts of the process while I got myself under control. I was instructed not to giggle anymore as the embryos were about to be inserted. This statement was enough to sober me up right away.

The doctor inserted the speculum and at the same time, the ultrasonographer moved the wand around my stomach until they had the view they were looking for. Two nurses were at my feet and they were using terminology that I had never heard before. One of them turned the lights to a minimal dim while the other handed swabs and other instruments to the doctor. Yet, even with all of this going on, this was a strangely, perfectly romantic experience. Mike stood next to me and held my hand tightly.

The doctor called for the embryologist who promptly came in with the catheter containing the two selected embryos. All at once Mike and I looked at the screen to see a little gray blip of fluid move out of the catheter and into place. "Perfect," the doctor said and the ultrasonographer pointed out for us the placement on the screen. We had witnessed a miracle. Maybe even two miracles. When the embryologist took the catheter to check that both embryos made it out successfully, we held our breaths. The news came that everything was clear and the army of hospital personnel left the room as efficiently as they entered.

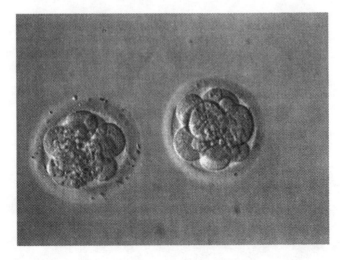

If there was any residual doubts about spending money, time, or emotional energy on an IVF cycle, this single moment cleared the fog. I understood all at once a love greater than I had ever known. These little gray blips on the screen were our future. They had the potential to bring us more happiness, frustration, gratitude and sadness than we could ever bring to each other in our lifetime. When the doctors had left the room and the lights were still out, I closed my eyes, placed a hand over my stomach and in my head I replayed a Peter, Paul and Mary song that my mom used to sing my sister and I when we were younger.

For Bobbie (Baby)

I'll walk in the rain by your side,
I'll cling to the warmth of your tiny hand.
I'll do anything to help you understand,
I'll love you more than anybody can.

And the wind will whisper your name to me,
Little birds will sing along in time,
The leaves will bow down when you walk by,
And morning bells will chime.

I'll be there when you're feeling down,
To kiss away the tears if you cry.
I'll share with you all the happiness I've found,
A reflection of the love in your eyes.

And I'll sing you the songs of the rainbow,
Whisper all the joy that is mine.
The leaves will bow down when you walk by,
And morning bells will chime.

Whoever these little embryos would be and whatever
lives they would touch, they were ours. We were theirs. We
may not have been present when they were conceived, and
it might not have happened the way we had dreamed when
we were first married, but we had created them and I
already knew I was in love with them.

Part Five: The Waiting Game

By this point in the cycle, I hope the infertiles reading
this are beginning to understand just how intense and

complicated the IVF cycle is. At each stage, a patient gives everything they have to ensure a positive outcome. They are invested in each injection and each ultrasound. The emotions build with every passing day. I found it remarkable that just when I thought my state of mind had held its full capacity of emotions, another step would take me to a place where I would continue to be tested, and like the steps prior, I would rise to the occasion.

Per order of my clinic, a specified number of days of "bed rest" were required following the embryo transfer. I had really looked forward to camping out on the couch and spending my day flipping through magazines, surfing the web, and watching movies. The problem was, as I was laying on the couch, the only thing that really had my attention was that I was actually carrying two little embryos whose potential for life was resting solidly on my shoulders, or at least my uterus.

I wondered what they were doing and what was happening inside of my body that I didn't know about. I talked to the embryos and oftentimes I'd rub my stomach gently. I prayed for them and smiled at the thought of them burrowing in and making a home for themselves for the next nine months. On the days when implantation should have been taking place I was especially anxious. I wished I had a camera in my uterus filming the whole thing like they do on those documentaries on the health channel.

It would be nice if these weeks were only filled with the excitement of anticipation, but the medication didn't stop just because my ovaries had fulfilled their end of the bargain. My uterus was next up at bat, and I had to take injections of progesterone to help the endometrial lining maintain a suitable environment for the embryos. Without the perfect lining in thickness and structure, the "textbook" embryos that we had created would not be able to implant.

Progesterone is the hormone that is produced by the body naturally after ovulation. With IVF, ovulation never actually occurs, because the eggs are retrieved just before this would actually happen. Therefore, the body of an IVF patient won't produce the levels of progesterone that could sustain a pregnancy should the embryos actually implant. Therefore, it's necessary to supplement with ongoing injections of progesterone.

After all of the injections in the stimulation phase of the cycle, I had become accustomed to the process of mixing meds and injecting them. I came to expect the initial sting and I didn't mind the extra minutes it took to prepare everything. Prior to actually performing this injection, I thought I was prepared for anything.

One of the unique aspects of the progesterone injection is that it is delivered intramuscularly. This one can't be given in the stomach. Instead, it must penetrate a muscle. In other words, this had to be delivered into my butt cheek area. The needle was longer than any of the others in order to make it through the layers of fat and into a muscle. Because of the location and size of the needle, I couldn't maneuver well enough to be able to hold the skin taut and inject the site at the same time. That meant Mike was the natural choice for the job.

A word from Mike:

By far the worst experience for me during the IVF cycle was having to give her the progesterone shots. The needle is an inch and a half long, and it's not a thin one either! I got one practice try while we were at the doctor's office. I watched as the nurse just pushed it in like it was nothing. Jenna winced, and for someone who had gained a fairly high threshold for pain, that was enough to make me nervous.

When it was time for me to do it for real, I failed miserably. As we were taught, Jenna bent over the sink in the bathroom and took the weight off of the side that we were going to inject. I imagine a dotted line bisecting her butt vertically and then horizontally, and selected the area the way I was shown. I held the skin down and tried to push the needle through her skin. It made an indent in the skin and it just wouldn't push through. I thought it was a dull needle, so I stopped and tried again. Finally, just when I was about to give up, it poked through completely. I ended up making her scream and curse. I thought the worst was over, but when I pulled the needle out a stream of bright red blood dribbled down her butt and pooled on her pajamas. Not a good start to a long career of injecting needles into my wife's rump!

I'm not sure which of us dreaded the nightly 8:00 p.m. routine more. I'd like to think it hurt me more than it hurt her, but judging by the bruises, I'd say that wasn't accurate. I never really got comfortable giving the shot, but we did get a system down. Jenna's face would be reflecting back at me in the mirror and I hated to see her with eyes shut in anticipation of what I was doing. I would try to block out her cursing as the needle went in. On the counter would be a warm facecloth and a swab to absorb the blood if I hit a bad spot. When it was over, I would use the warm cloth to rub the oil around.

By then it was only 23 hours and 55 minutes until we had to do it all over again.

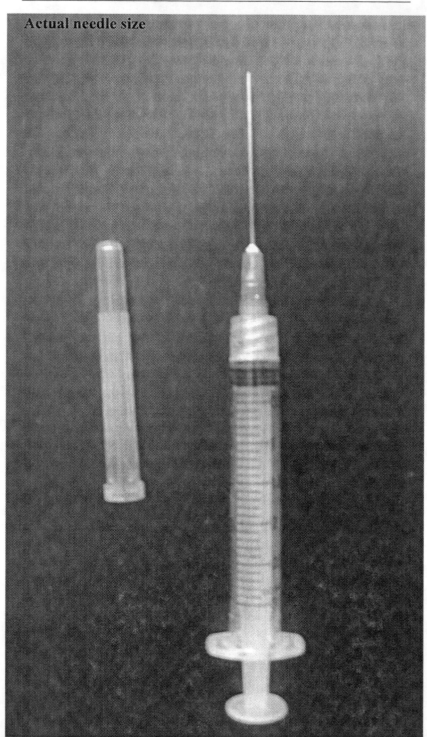

Actual needle size

The other peculiarity of this medication is that it comes in the form of oil. This means the consistency of it is thick and can coagulate upon injection. A lot of IVF patients and professionals have researched the best methods of delivering the medication to avoid it clumping under the skin, but no matter what we tried, I would end up with a cotton ball sized knot at the area of injection. We used a warm wet facecloth to heat the oil and syringe, we rubbed the area prior to and after the injection to distribute the oil, and we tried a heating pad after injecting. Nothing seemed to work any wonders. Each night Mike changed sides to give the one cheek time to recuperate. Inevitably, by the time we were about five or six days into the shots, I was all done sitting comfortably.

The bruises that swelled around the injection sites became one more daily reminder of what my body was going through, but the progesterone left other marks as well. The possible side effects of this one medication included breast tenderness, bloating, tiredness, nausea, mood swings, and headaches. Combined with the weight gain and constipation I was already experiencing, I was a real joy to be around.

I am wondering if there are any fertiles reading this who are thinking, "Hey, constipation, fatigue, bloating, sore enlarged breasts... those all sound like pregnancy symptoms." That's right. The massive dose of progesterone in the shot form has a tendency to produce the same symptoms as a woman who is, in fact, pregnant. In my case, my progesterone level was 90 just days after the little embryos should have been implanting. A progesterone level of 90 is somewhere around the 28th week of pregnancy for the average woman.

One of the cruelest parts to the IVF cycle is the experience during the two weeks while waiting for the pregnancy test. While a couple is praying for a positive result, their body is effectively giving them every reason to believe they will achieve that. When a normally fertile woman is pregnant, she would most likely never have a single symptom during these weeks, and yet the infertile ironically experiences many side effects masked as symptoms throughout this time.

It is simply agonizing to wake up to a barrage of pregnancy symptoms one morning and by later in the day they are gone, only to be followed by another wave of possibility the next day.

Tuesday, June 21, 2005
Twinges and Pains; My Imaginary Friends

I feel like I've been plowed down by a steamroller. Today I returned to work, field day no less, and even though I really spent most of the day sitting down, it was totally exhausting. The schedule was insane with only two 20 minute breaks and 36 kids running through every 20 minutes.

Around noon I starting feeling some really sharp pains in my abdomen and of course, I started thinking that maybe it was implantation or other signs that I might be pregnant. But now they are gone and it's almost like I have to try hard to remember them. I wonder if I'm making up these feelings or reading too much into normal feelings that I otherwise would never have noticed.

I find myself crying at the drop of a hat. Am I reading into that as well? I know the progesterone shots can act as exaggerated PMS, and yet, even these bursts of emotion give me hope. Every moment is filled with hope and anxiety, frustration and anticipation. I never know how I feel or what to do to make myself feel better. I hate feeling so out of control of myself and yet if these are the symptoms of pregnancy, I will gladly succumb to them for the next nine months.

What makes me think this isn't working is that all of the side effects of the progesterone that I would want to consider "symptoms" are beginning to go away. Last night I was able to sleep on my stomach without my boobs killing me as they did the nights before. I didn't feel as nauseous as I have for the past few days. I wonder if the progesterone is fading and my body is resuming normal functioning.

This is the worst of the waiting I've experienced in these years of trying to have a baby. I think it's because this is the closest we've ever come... and yet I so desperately hope it isn't the closest we will ever come!

I feel myself sitting in the middle of a seesaw; torn between wanting to know and wanting to revel in being "a little pregnant". I am anxious to find my way through this weekend and come out whole on the other side. I have no idea how this is going to go. Sometimes the glimmers of hope and optimism make me certain that we will have happy news for the first time. At these times there is a peace of mind that comes, which is amazing. I could live in those moments. As long as we are waiting for the moment of truth, there is a hope that comforts me and gives me happiness. As much as I often want to just know the answers and be done with this turmoil, there is a something wonderful about having possibility. Am I really so ready to give that up? Maybe I could just keep taking the progesterone injections and see what happens in the next few months... that way I don't ever have to really get the news... unless it's good, and then I want it tomorrow! What a nutcase I am!

Part Six: The Pregnancy Test

The days crawled along as a snail's pace. Both Mike and I were torn between wanting to know the answer and afraid to lose the adrenaline of anticipation. I felt certain that I would have some kind of instinctual feeling if I were pregnant, but Mike's optimism kept me going on a more hopeful path. He would say, "We can test today or we can test tomorrow, but the answer will still be the same. It just depends on when you want to find out that you're pregnant." I both loved and loathed those words. If he was right, he was going to happily gloat for the rest of our lives over how he knew all along. But if he was wrong, I was going to have to watch the joy on the face of the man I loved more than anything in this world dissipate into disappointment.

Saturday, June 25, 2005
The Verdict is in...

Apparently my life sentence in infertility hell will not be commuted any time soon.

At 5:00 a.m. we dipped the sticks into a cup of urine. As soon as we unwrapped the tests, I immediately regretted it. I walked back into the bedroom, leaving Mike by himself in the bathroom. I watched his expression intently as he looked down at the counter. I wanted to will it to be positive. Three minutes later, he was still standing there. If it had been positive he would have come right out. I knew that, but I want to believe he was trying to surprise me or was gathering his thoughts and figuring out how to tell me the good news. The seconds and minutes went by and I knew the truth. I didn't want him to face me. Finally, after five minutes, I said, "The time is up." He turned out the bathroom light and I just burst into tears. Without a word, he hugged me. It wasn't the type of hug you give after a long day at work. It was the deep soulful way you grasp only your spouse in the moment when you realize you love them beyond reason, beyond fear, beyond doubt and sadness.

The truth was obvious, but as I cried I had to ask anyway, still hoping maybe there was a mistake. There were two tests on the counter. One even glared, "NOT PREGNANT". Guess that one was unmistakable. There was no way to hold the one at different angles and pretend otherwise. Mike said when he looked at the test he actually thought it read, "Fuck You"... what a slap in the face. He was so right. I couldn't have said it better myself. I laughed. I don't anticipate laughing like that for a while.

I've cried uncontrollably for hours. I couldn't hold myself together and the emotions seemed so much rawer that I had anticipated. We went for a walk on the beach for a couple hours and cried some more as I watched a woman running down the boardwalk with her jogging stroller. That won't be me. Not this year. We came home. Mike went to bed and hasn't gotten out since. I tried to sleep, but I found myself staring at my ceiling fan, and crying some more.

The really awful part is that I'm not even sure it's completely hit me yet. Right now I feel numb.

Mike still thinks the blood test will be positive, but we aren't talking about that. I told him I can't handle having to face this twice, so I need to deal with as much of the pain as I can now. He understood and has been really wonderful about holding me and hugging me, and letting me cry as much as I need to. I think the news from the beta tomorrow will hurt him more than me.

I can't help but think of what we'd be doing right now if it had turned out positive. The idea that we might be out driving around telling people the news, or that we would have walked on the beach and talked about names and dreams is heartbreaking. That happiness was so close. I had it in my sights. I could feel it if I tried hard enough, and now it seems so far away.

I became so much more attached to them than I thought I had. They were there. They were healthy and viable. They were the perfect sizes and shapes. They had divided perfectly. Then they were just gone. I don't understand it. I don't know why this would have happened. How did I go from being the mom of twins to being just another failed cycle in the span of three minutes?

I can spin through my mind a million moments of when they decided not to make a home in me and it kills me to think that I might have done something wrong. Was it the day of the transfer when I lifted my leg to put on the sock? Did I get up too many times to go to the bathroom? Was the shower too hot ? Was it because I got mad at the dog and raised my voice when he pooped in the house? Was it because I was bending over to pick the poop up when no one was home to do it? Was chocolate ice cream too cold? Did we not get enough progesterone in the one time when some of it came out? Did I not put the Estrace in far enough? Or did the embryos just decide to not even try?

I don't know what to think right now. I don't even know how to think.

When the final results of the blood pregnancy test come in, it really doesn't matter if I had taken five, one, or zero home tests in the days that preceded that phone call. The pain is so intense and indescribable. There is no preparation for the news that once again I have lost the fight. I might have said to a half dozen people that I 'knew' it was negative. But the fact is, no matter how much I knew it to be true, even if I was 99.9% certain of a negative, there is 100% of me praying deeply to be wrong. The .1% of me that wasn't certain always overpowers the rest. The calling to parent is more intense than any home test or gut feeling can account for.

The phone rings. I wait for the second ring to catch the caller ID. I know who it is. I wait for another ring. *These seconds will change my life. Whatever the answer is, everything will be different in the next 30 seconds.*

Hello? *This is it. Brace yourself, Jenna. You already know the answer, but you might be wrong... no, no don't do that to yourself, you know the answer. Don't expect anything different..*

May I speak to Jenna?

This is. *Just say it. No, don't say it. Oh for God's sake, stop torturing yourself. Listen. She sounds sad. Listen.*

This is ***** from the clinic.
Are these seconds, minutes or hours that are passing? This is no time to inhale lady, just say it. I already know anyway. You have that tone....

I wish I had better news. You need to stop the injections blah blah... stop the estrace... blah blah ... wait for a period.... *I hear nothing more than broken sentences. I hear the sound of emptiness; my heart pounding in an empty body. There is hollowness in my soul and the ache in my heart explodes to my throat. Just get me off the phone. It's too hard. I can't do this again.*

Part Seven: Grieving

There are many misunderstood aspects to infertility, but this part of the process is most painful when it's expressed inappropriately by someone who, though perfectly well-intentioned, is misguided. Hopefully if you've read this carefully, you can see how personally invested an infertile couple will necessarily become in the process. It's not a physical or emotional or financial commitment. Infertility is all of the above, not to mention oftentimes spiritual as well. Infertiles give themselves, body, mind and soul, to the experience and in the event of a failed cycle, the mourning process can only be compared to the death of the closest loved one.

In the days following this first IVF failure, everything was a blur. I had a difficult time getting myself to the shower or off the couch. Not only was I emotionally exhausted, but my body was feeling the effects of a crash in hormones. With my head pounding from a migraine and my body preparing to expel the remnants of the entire cycle through a period, I was as drained as I had ever been. I don't think I realized how involved I had become until it was actually over and the medications were flushing out of my system.

What made this experience increasingly difficult was the fact that what Mike and I had lost couldn't completely be explained to anyone around us. We were alone in our sadness. No one had met these would-be babies but us. We had seen them in their more fragile and basic structures. It may sound strange, but I had reveled in their possibility and now I was grieving their loss.

To those who cared for us, it was a failed cycle and there could be another cycle around the corner to look forward to. A failed cycle was a reason to have some drinks and eat a lot of junk food. The statue of limitations of being sad is short in their minds. It should be relatively easy to move on and formulate another plan of action. I found that most people who knew of our struggles would say they were sorry and in the same sentence they'd ask, "What are you going to do next?" I couldn't think about the next few minutes, never mind the next two months.

We tried to enjoy not being on medications and not

having to worry about the next monitoring session, but these things had become aspects of our life that, in a strange way, were comforting in their own way. Without them, there was no possibility to be pregnant, and I would have gladly traded away my freedom to enjoy the luxuries of alcohol for the intoxication of hope. I experienced several stages of grief as the actuality of our situation came into view. I went through periods of denial, anger, numbness and depression, acceptance, and finally, I was ready to walk back into social functioning and the routine of everyday living.

Even though I knew in reality that the nurse who called with our results wasn't mistaken, in the moments following the official news of the failure, I wanted desperately to believe that they had ordered the wrong blood test or accidentally called the wrong person. I refused to face the knowledge that the last two months were all for nothing. I wanted to continue taking the progesterone shots and be retested in a few days. When someone called to see how things were going, I couldn't utter the answer that my mind knew, but my heart refused to accept.

The transition to anger was quick. I distinctly remember walking the dog in the same afternoon when we learned the news from the nurse. Suddenly, my pace quickened and I broke into a run. I hadn't run in months. I had been told not to do any cardiovascular activity to ensure that I didn't lose any weight. Here I was, pulling my little Lhasa Apso, Fenway, up a steep hill as fast as I could. I was fueled entirely by the frustration and infuriation of the lost cycle. As I ran, my anger raged with memories of futile shots and imaginary pregnancy symptoms that I convinced myself were the real thing. I hated myself for talking to the embryos as if they were our babies just days earlier when the reality was they had already dissolved into the tissues of

---

my uterus. I felt stupid for thinking that I could change our situation with meditation.

I was cleaning out the bathroom laboratory later the next morning when I suddenly started to sob inexcusably. As I tossed out the empty vials of medications and wiped down the counter, I felt as if I was cleaning up the remainder of my future. There began the stage of depression. I fear that I remained in this place the longest. For days I avoided contact with anyone who called or came by the house. I found myself showering several times a day just to have something to do, as if the heat of the shower would cleanse the pain I was feeling. In public, the sadness took on a numbing sensation. It showed itself as isolation from everyone and everything. I felt incredibly disconnected to the world around me. People joked around me and I would half chuckle as if I were present, but I knew my heart was miles away.

Wednesday, June 29, 2005
So Far Away From the Finish Line

I thought I was doing better and starting to move on, but today I'm right back where I was on Saturday. I'm seeing this failure as losing something more than some blood and tissue. I have never felt farther away from the goal than when I get my period and I see all of our work literally being flushed down the toilet. Everything we've wanted and dreamed about seems so far away right now; so utterly impossible.

I've pretty much secluded myself from everything and everyone. What could they say that will make any of this better? They won't understand and they won't see it for what it is. For them, they probably think this is routine at this point. They will see it as just another cycle down the tubes, not the loss of two babies that were ours; two little lives that we saw in their earliest stages. They'll try futilely to pep talk me into not being sad and trying to move on, when the fact of the matter is, there is nothing that will make any of this okay. They'll think I'm being dramatic and that I'm making this bigger than it is.

So, talking to people about this seems like a waste of time. I'm lonely and scared that this is the end of the road for us and there is nothing that can change that for me. Having to explain the technical aspects of this isn't for me right now, not to mention the fact that the initial, "how are you doing?" question is something I'm having a hard time answering for myself. Do I say "fine" just to move on, or do I tell them the truth and have to listen to all of their ignorant, inane advice on dealing with something they cannot begin to comprehend.

The advice has been pouring in from family and friends to which I have several responses that I don't dare utter out loud.

"Don't worry, it'll happen when it's meant to"... *So am I meant to go broke and suffer through 776 days of infertility hell?*

(here's an original one) "Just take a deep breath, relax and look out the window"... *Why? Is there a baby out there that I can have?*

"You have to do whatever it takes."... *So what does it take? Because I thought it took some sperm and an egg, but I just fertilized 16 of those and I still don't have anything.*

This is my typical defense... sarcasm. Rather than letting people in, I push them away. I chalk it up to the easy answer of "they can't possibly understand." But what do I do to help them understand? Nothing. I've got enough jobs right now.

Summer break had started and without the vitality of my students to help me stay focused on progress, I fell into a pit of despondency for which there seemed no reason to revive myself. I moved dispassionately through the days waiting for something to change. I disengaged from everything and everyone, and remained that way until I literally got bored of the monotony of myself.

The day came when I woke up and decided that I needed to not waste time wallowing in the rejection I was feeling. I logged on to my computer and began researching what I could have done better. At the time, I thought this was an incredibly mature and proactive step to take. I prided myself on my determination and was ready to put the past behind me and learn from the mistakes we had made. In reality, this was just me trying to make a deal with a higher power. If I promised to not have even caffeine free soda or if I vowed to do acupuncture, or if I worked hard on not getting worked up about every monitoring result... the list went on. The problem that I would later learn was that the more deals I made, the more responsibility I personally took for each failure. The promises I made were virtually impossible to maintain and when a cycle didn't work, I would have only myself to blame.

Lastly, I was able to accept the reality of our recent failed cycle and begin to move into transitioning back into a life where I had friendships and family, and fun things to look forward to. Mike and I had been through a hellish couple of months, not to mention a few years that were borderline abominable as far as our family building plans were concerned. We wanted to do something for ourselves that had nothing to do with infertility. A vacation was one idea, but that just seemed too cliché and besides, we had a home that still needed furnishing. We decided it would be a positive step if we took some money and furnished one of the many empty rooms. Not only would it be something to make us feel like our dreams for that home would eventually come true, but to be frivolous with a few dollars was something that we needed to do to feel normal again.

Chapter 5

Rationalizing the Irrational

Anyone who loves an infertile will necessarily ask the obvious question. Why keep going? Just stop. This seems like the obvious answer. Watching an infertile go through the pain of a lost cycle time and time again can be heartbreaking. Move on. Isn't that the most rational idea? Perhaps. But nothing about this disease is rational. What I have is infertility. It is not just a disease of the body. It affects the very nature of who I am at the core of my soul. Never give up. Never give in. That was how I lived all other aspects of my life. It was what I had been taught; if you try hard enough, and want it bad enough, anything is possible. How many of us have heard, "If at first you don't succeed, try, try again." This was what I taught my students. Anyone can give in, but the strength of one's character is only tested when times are tough. It was something I believed beyond all of the failures.

Sometimes it can even feel like an addiction.

The gambler's fallacy: The mistaken belief that past

events will affect future events when dealing with random activities. In the case of infertility, it is the notion that an event is more likely to occur simply because it has not happened in a long time. In other words, the more you play the game, the better your odds are that it will work.

Long before we ever adopted the title of "infertile", Mike and I had made the decision to never give up and never give in. That was how we worked as a team through all of the challenges we faced prior to our marriage. There was, however, one, and only one, time prior to our struggles with infertility when both of us were ready to throw in the towel on a situation. The lesson was a vicarious one; something we learned in the adult's playground of Las Vegas, Nevada; a place where the gambler's fallacy was lived every minute of every day.

When Mike and I had money for vacations, one of the places where we had a tremendous amount of fun was Vegas. On our first trip, we brought a friend with us. This friend had a system that he had calculated out on paper and worked through countless times with his mathematical father prior to even getting on the plane. He believed that if he played the same two numbers on the roulette board and increased his bet at every interval, then within a certain number of plays he would be guaranteed to win. The earlier he won, the greater the profit, but regardless of when he won, he believed he could not lose.

On our first night in Vegas, he and Mike headed to the tables. Our friend, with a few thousand dollars in his pocket to spend, began the system. He concentrated on the two green numbers: "0" and "00". He sat patiently at the table while other players came and went. Each time the ball spun around, he waited, flipping chips between his fingers and confident that he was going to win. Time and time again, people won and screamed for joy, or left the table, tail between their legs and feeling forlorn that their lucky numbers didn't hit. Dealers came and went, and came back again. But our friend, hours into play, still sat there, having not won, but comfortable that it would be any time.

With only two plays left, the little metal ball whirled around and around the mechanism. In those seconds my heart was sinking and my eyes were closed. I couldn't believe he had been sitting there for hours and playing the same two numbers. Not once had they come up while other numbers had been called a half dozen times. The ball bounced around the numbers until finally it landed on yet another number that was not his. A thought echoed in my mind that my parents had shared. It was easy to get caught up in thinking you could beat the game, but Vegas wouldn't be Vegas if the odds weren't in the casino's favor. I'm sure these casino employees had seen people like our friend before. They probably spent their coffee breaks talking about the last poor sap to get sucked into the myth of a system.

With still a bit of money left, Mike and I tried to convince him to leave. He still had enough money to have a good time for the week and we didn't want him to start our vacation broke. He refused. He maintained that he had to play the system the entire way through. I felt sick to my stomach with dread.

And wouldn't you know, his number came up: "00". It couldn't have been a better ending if it were fiction. He had actually won. On the last possible spin, the little metal nemesis became his very best friend. Mike and I had lost faith in the system. Looking back on it, I cringe at the thought of what it would have been like to pull off of the plan and stand by as that last spin took place. What would we have felt when we realized that had we just stuck it out, we would have won? If you were in this situation, how would you have felt?

I think about that experience in comparison to our journey through infertility. In so many ways it mirrors the patience, the false belief in a system, and the fear of walking away from the potential big win just before it was about to hit. We kept going on the infertility journey because we didn't know what was around the next corner. We could imagine the miracle that we would be denying ourselves if we didn't see it through to an end.

"So why not walk away?" asks the fertile. "Why not cut your losses now?" I suppose it's the belief that our number might be next. We want to believe that with each change in protocol and every prayer from loved ones, something will make the difference. We hear stories of couples who went through half a dozen rounds of treatment or more and nothing ever worked. Then finally on the last round, when they were about to throw in the towel, on the last spin of the wheel, they hit the jackpot. Their number came up and they were blessed with a healthy and beautiful family.

I suppose I can understand why it would be difficult for a person who never desired children to empathize with infertility. It would be like me trying to understand the drive to climb to the top of the corporate ladder. As a teacher, that's just not my ambition. The more removed from the yearning, the harder it is to feel the connection.

But what is difficult to digest is the lack of understanding from those who actually have children. As much as I believe 'they can never really get it,' I feel like they should be near the top of the list of those handing out compassion. Most people who have kids will claim they would do anything for them, that they wouldn't give them up for all the money in our world. Infertiles feel exactly the same. The difference is, for the fertile these are somewhat empty words. As much as they claim they would do or pay anything, they've never really been asked to cough up the price to parent. Where the infertiles are concerned, these convictions are challenged at every new cycle, and at every step we rise to those promises. We WOULD do anything, and often we DO spend all of the money in our world.

Chapter 6

The Biggest Present Under the Christmas Tree is Just an Empty Box

There was a time when we thought we had won the jackpot for all infertiles; the Holy Grail of IVF. We had gambled on this cycle and put ourselves into debt hoping that due to the percentages we were given, success would be found in our favor. The magic number was 2.1. We had been told that 2.1 was the average number of IVF cycles that it took to achieve pregnancy at our clinic. This was cycle number two. We were still amateurs in the IVF arena and did not plan on becoming veterans.

I employed every tactic I had read about. I was doing yoga, meditation and this time, acupuncture. The extra $80 per week I spent on this was another bill that we would be haunted by, but if it was the one thing that could possibly make a difference, it was worth trying. Once or twice per week I was lying on a table, surrounded by the sounds of nature playing on a CD, and trying to be as still as possible while my acupuncturist inserted approximately 20 needles thinner than the thinnest pin into my ears, scalp, toes, legs, wrists and abdomen. I didn't find this to be 45 minutes of relaxation that others felt.

Little strands of hair would find their way out of my ponytail and tickled my cheeks. I would wriggle my nose to itch it away the best I could. Instead of going into a meditative state, I would be looking around the room at the posters of acupuncture points and studying the ceiling tiles. On the occasions when I lay on my stomach, I would feel the discomfort of my sinuses filling up from allergies and I'd spend the minutes picturing the cement of mucus settling in and making a home in my head. It wasn't the ideal way to spend an hour, or $80, but if it meant I wouldn't be later wondering, "what if", it was worth it.

Thursday, July 14, 2005
Hoping on Pins and Needles

Last night my infertility treatments took a totally different course as I experienced my first acupuncture appointment. I'm not sure if this will be the thing that makes me all better and brings a baby to us, but it's definitely worth a shot... or should I say, a needle?

When I walked into the office, I immediately knew this was going to be a different experience from what I was used to. Instead of the stuffy doctor's office, there were wind chimes in the waiting room and the magazines on the table weren't *Time* or *Entertainment Weekly*, they were all about yoga and meditation. I sat in a wicker chair instead of the metal cushioned ones I knew so well, and I looked out real windows at real flowers instead of the prints on the wall of my clinic.

The woman who did this, Lindsay, was really a sweet and wonderful woman. She told me about her own experiences with infertility and how acupuncture helped her; inspiring her to do this for other women. I was really nervous at first and tried to put on a happy face, but it wasn't more than a few minutes before she figured that was a cover for how I was feeling, and soon I found myself stunned by how insightful she was.

She took my pulse on both wrists and checked my tongue. Weird... Then she started to get animated and said that she had "all kinds of lights going off" and felt like she could really help me. She did say that my type of infertility was one of the most difficult to deal with, especially in the 4-6 weeks we have before it's time to do the next retrieval. Nonetheless, she said she was happy to give it a try and that she wanted me to start on some herbs right away. Then she started the process of performing the acupuncture.

It was strange and a little uncomfortable, but I can see how in a few more sessions I'll be able to relax and possibly enjoy it. A few of the needles hurt, but most of them just made me feel like I didn't want to move for fear of screwing things up. One of the needles was actually very painful. It felt different from all the others. As soon as she put it into the inside of my wrist, I felt a sharp pain and a burning sensation up my arm. I really thought she had done something wrong and when I asked her about it, she started to laugh. She said, "That one is the connection to your uterus." So apparently, my uterus is truly equal opportunity when it comes to rejecting people. HA!

At any rate, I've made an appointment for next Wednesday. With this first one behind me, I'm anxious to see if this will really have an impact on the rest of me, as well as the issues with infertility. I've spoken with the nurse at my clinic and she said the herbs were perfectly fine to take, so as of tonight I'll be popping nine pills in addition to the rest of my protocol.

Unfortunately, the cycle immediately started out worse than any we had done previously. On several occasions we were faced with the possibility of having the whole cycle cancelled. It was a dread that most infertile women face at some point; never making it to the egg retrieval, which means weeks of the process had gone by and the patience I withstood through the birth control pills and the beginning week of the injections might have all been for not.

My hormone levels were uncooperative, fluctuating for no apparent reason, and the ultrasound showed a dominant follicle; one egg as opposed to the dozen or so that would be ideal. The option that faced us was to convert the IVF cycle into an IUI cycle, reducing the success rate considerably. We had done a number of IUI cycles and knew this was not a realistic possibility for us.

We were determined to see the cycle through to an end. For better or worse, the IVF had to continue. The decision was made to let the dominant follicle go and concentrate on building up the smaller ones. The medications and dosages were changed, and we managed to squeak up to the day of the egg retrieval. I felt like I had dodged a bullet. We made it to a place where at least there was a possibility of a pregnancy even though it was remote. In my mind, the quality of the eggs they retrieved was not going to be anything to brag about, but at least there was a chance. To my surprise, they managed to retrieve 19 eggs. I was astounded with the great news. One more hurdle overcome. The next step was to see how many fertilized.

The next day, as I was recovering from the retrieval procedure, I received the phone call that 16 of the eggs had fertilized. Things were starting to turn around in our favor. But still, we had been down a similar road before, and I held my heart in check. Fertilization was not our issue. There were still no guarantees that anything would be different. The quality of those 16 embryos was debatable, and we would have to wait 48 hours until the transfer day to see if they were still growing.

Two days later we were back at the hospital bright and early, and with a full bladder waiting to make a home for the embryos that were selected. I had only taken half of the valium dose so I could be a better participant in the transfer. With bated breath we awaited the embryologist's news as to the quality of the embryos we had.

When our doctor came in, he held a clipboard close to his chest. His expression was in stark contrast to last transfer where he was smiling and excited. Immediately, I knew something was wrong. Standing next to the embryologist, they explained that the embryo cells were still multiplying, but that they were not the quality they had hoped. In an instant my heart sank. Mike squeezed my hand as we listened to them discuss the possibility of transferring three embryos.

My heart sank deeper. We had discussed this option early into my treatment. When we initiated the conversation about IVF, I had wanted to transfer three embryos right away in order to increase my odds of success. Our reproductive endocrinologist had clearly repeated that triplets would be a tremendous risk to me and the babies, and that he would personally consider triplets to be a failure. There was no room for negotiations on this. He further explained that to transfer three embryos was only a consideration in a situation where there was a limited chance for pregnancy or in cases of advanced maternal age. I was 29. Clearly my issue was the former. It rang through my brain like a freight train… "limited chance for pregnancy".

After the transfer was completed, I laid in the hospital bed holding Mike's hand and feeling that familiarity of defeat make a comfortable nest in my heart. I knew it would be there for a while. I didn't go home and dream of nursery colors or sing any songs in my heart. Instead, I slept on the couch for a day or so and then continued my normal August routine of preparing for another school year. I didn't even feel badly about not taking the required number of bed rest days. *What was the point anymore?*

As the days stretched on, I felt nothing different from the previous cycles and the certainty of failure rested heavy on my heart. My acupuncturist had insisted that she felt a "slippery pulse" which could indicate pregnancy. I was feeling elated. The news had come regarding the other embryos that were not selected and my elation turned to defeat.

Saturday, August 20, 2005
Ambivalent With a Side of Pissed

Last night we got the mail and saw the fertilization report that was done on the day of the transfer. It couldn't have been more disappointing. Out of the 19 eggs and the 16 embryos, and the 13 that we left there to mature, none, absolutely none of them grew to the freezing state. Even in our past failed cycle there were four that were frozen.

So at that point any optimism that was still left from the acupuncture appointment was lost. What are the chances that they just happened to pick the right one, two and three embryos that wouldn't have died? I went to bed and had one of the worst night's sleeps I've had in a very long time. Every conscious or subconscious fear turned itself into a dream; from realizing this IVF didn't work, to my father being attacked by bees, to my classroom being out of control. It was stress after stress.

I should have known that waking up wasn't going to be any better. Mike nudged me awake at 7 a.m. and wanted to take a

99

pregnancy test. I really didn't want to, but I agreed just to take it and he could see it if he didn't let me know what it said. I just didn't want to keep taking the progesterone shots for the next few days knowing it was futile. Naturally though, the fact that he was standing there for so long just showed it didn't work. When he jumped in the shower, I pulled the test from the garbage and looked. Clearly negative.

I'm not really that sad yet, just disappointed. I had that feeling of the outcome for a while, so I'm not surprised, but it is always an unpredictable feeling when you see it for real. There was no crying this time, but I'm not ruling it out. We've got four more progesterone shots to humor and now that we've taken one test, we may end up just taking the other three that are left between now and Wednesday. There's nothing like being kicked in the face a few more times.

I'm glad we did the test now. At least I can start dealing with the results now instead of the day before school starts. I'm going to get the house cleaned up, clean my car, and start thinking about the new stuff I'm going to do with the kids this year. I have to work on getting myself back into shape and preparing myself for whatever life has to offer.

Mike was very supportive after I told him I looked at the test. He did the usual barrage of reasons why it might not be accurate, and then I just looked at him dead in the eyes and said more seriously than before, "It's not murky and you know it. It's negative. It's just negative." I didn't want to break his optimism, but I knew it was too easy to convince ourselves that if we held the test up just right, or looked at it long enough, we could make up a new ending to the story. After that I think he understood that it was the real thing and it wasn't going to do either of us any good to over think it or pretend that the obvious was a lie. Next we went into planning mode and decided that we would do the consult with our doctor to find out what he thinks happened, and then we'd make an appointment with the satellite office of another clinic just to see what they think we should do. Probably around December we'll do the frozen ones (Mike wants to try one more fresh) and then we are done for good. He says if all of that is negative, we should go to Aruba for one of my vacation weeks and then start researching other opportunities.

Days passed and each day we took another test. Each time it came up negative. My acupuncturist was certain there was something "going on in there" even after I explained the results of the two other pregnancy tests I had taken since the first. The struggle in my heart of wanting to believe in her versus needing to protect myself from what seemed like eventual heartbreak was overwhelming.

Not wanting to put Mike through another round of disappointment, I took another test when he wasn't home. Fifteen minutes after the test was in the garbage, I pulled it back out. To my shock, there was an extremely thin line, but only when I held it at an angle. In my mind I knew there was reason that the directions said any results that appeared after three minutes were invalid. Logically, I understood that this was most likely an evaporation line. Still, my acupuncturist's words kept repeating in my mind, "I've got my story, and I'm sticking to it." I wanted so badly to believe the nightmare was over. I called the clinic and begged them to move up the official pregnancy blood test a day.

Tuesday, August 23, 2005
The Longest 15 Minutes of My Life

This morning, the nurse said I could call the office around 11:30 for the results of the pregnancy test. I thought I wanted the results. I thought I needed to know for sure if I am falsely pinning my hopes and heart to a faint gray line on a home pregnancy test, and the words of an "alternative healer". I went to school to take my mind off of this, which did seem to work for a little while, but I had to rush home all of a sudden because I felt like I was going to explode with diarrhea.

If there is a baby in there, I'm certainly not making it a very nice home at the moment.

It's 11:26 and with four minutes to go.

It's 11:29, one more minute.

It's 11:30 and I'm trying to wait as long as I can. I don't want to lose this feeling of elation and anxiety. I have never been this high in my life and to think it might come crashing down is too much to bear. To think that every dream I've had for the last three years is a phone call away is unbearably frightening.

I thought I wanted to surprise Mike, but now, more than any surprise, I just wish he was here and that we could go through this together. He would call for me and no matter the answer, I wouldn't be alone.

It's 11:36 and it would be over by now if I could just get myself off of the couch. I feel paralyzed. I think the last five minutes went by and I forgot to breathe.

Okay Jenna, just do it. Just make the call. You have to deal with this one way or the other.

Okay, here I go. I'm going.

It's 11:40. I made the call and they are very busy so they have to call me back. Seriously? This is the rest of my life and they have to call me back.

▪▪▪

12:39

So it's official. I'm pregnant. *Did I just say that? ME?* I'm pregnant? *Oh my God. I have to look at those words again.*

I'm pregnant, I'm pregnant, I'm pregnant, I'm pregnant, I'm pregnant!

My HCG level is 91 and they consider anything over 50 to be pregnant. The nurse said 91 is a good starting number, even though to me it feels like it's on the low side. Nonetheless, I will be happy with this number as it is the first time I've even had a number to even consider.

I asked about the possibility of twins or triplets, and she said she doesn't go there with patients at this point because anything is possible. But I looked it up, because that's what I do, and it seems that it is below the norm for even a single pregnancy.

I just have to enjoy this moment. I have never felt it before. I will never feel another first moment like this again and I have to relish it for everything it's worth.

I called Mike and wanted to scream the news, but I held it to myself. He's coming home for a late lunch and I can't wait to tell him the news that he is going to be a father. Wow, I can't believe I just typed that. I can't help but smile.

After I hung up the phone it was so strangely silent in the house. With the screaming and excitement in my own head, it feels odd that there is nothing but silence around me. I walked into the spare room and for the first time, I could see, without sadness, what it was meant to be. The stripes I had painted on the wall when we first moved in, and the fabric swatches I had collected for drapes and blankets, all finally had meaning. It wasn't abstract; it wasn't remote. It wasn't a dream far away. I walked into the room and felt I would remember that moment forever. It was the first time our baby would be in its room and in our home.

I'm pregnant, I'm pregnant, I'm pregnant, I'm pregnant, I'm pregnant!

There are no words that could possibly express the kind of emotion felt by an infertile who is able to finally feel the joy of being pregnant. For so long my body was empty.

The echo in my heart had banged against my chest for years and finally it felt enveloped in the softest, warmest blanket I could know. I fell in love with the bundle of cells that were made in a laboratory and placed in me. They had beaten the odds of a horrible cycle and miraculously nestled into an environment that seemed to reject every other opportunity for life. I admired the strength of the baby that we had created and in the first minutes after learning the news of my pregnancy, I promised to nurture and protect it with every ounce of love and strength I could muster.

A word from Mike:

It was a typical day with the same routines, but I could just sense something was about to happen. I ended up getting a call from Jenna around 1:00 p.m. asking what time I was coming home. As I drove home, I was trying to prepare myself for some bad news. Although it wasn't official, the pregnancy test we took a few days earlier confirmed that the second round of IVF didn't work. I was nervous that I was about to hear some more bad news or that Jenna was having a really hard time digesting the newest failure. As I walked around to the back of the house, Jenna was standing at the top of the deck. It was at that moment that I knew she was pregnant.

It was absolutely impossible for her to conceal her excitement. I thought I would play along with her and let her tell me. I definitely knew though. About halfway up the stairs, she blurted out that she was pregnant. She obviously couldn't hold the news in for very long! It was a crazy feeling as I tried to soak it in. There were so many thoughts that went through my mind simultaneously as I climbed the last steps to get to her. Is this really going to happen? We had been through so many disappointments over the last few years that it was very hard to believe the quest was finally over. I felt an immediate urge to ensure that Jenna was safe and secure. I thought about purchasing a safer car and adding a security system to the house. I also wondered how we were going to afford raising a child. This feeling, however, went away very quickly after thinking about how much we had already spent with the various infertility procedures. Having a child at this point was going to give us a raise!!

I think the most prominent memory I have of that day is watching Jenna gently touching her stomach. There just wasn't anything more satisfying than watching the woman I loved care for our child.

Despite what people might think, infertility doesn't end when pregnancy is achieved. Many infertiles, such as myself, find that in the midst of their excitement, a pervading feeling of uncertainty clouds the reality of success. Like many infertile women, I was overwhelmed with news of the pregnancy, but cautious of my heart. We had traveled a long and arduous road and the emotions of potential calamity were in direct conflict with the sheer amazement of a future we had neatly tucked away in our minds.

Sharing the news of our success felt like a present I wanted to give over and over again. The people who had stood by us for so long, those who had provided support during the difficult times and those who had provided partial funding for the cycles, had felt the anxiety that we had, only on a different level. I felt responsible for their disappointment time and time again. I had yearned for a time when I could be the source of good news instead of bad. Finally that moment was ours and we wanted to make it as special as possible.

To be able to present them with this news were moments to savor. I created presents for each to open; a framed poem for each of our parents which could be replaced with ultrasound pictures and swapped out for pictures of birthdays and Christmases to come; and a counting book for our nephew containing the number of days until his cousin arrived. Each experience of sharing our news released more of the burden of infertility. I knew it would always be with me, but I began to feel relief with each day.

Being pregnant changed a lot of my outlook. I felt a relief that I could get pregnant, but the actuality of being pregnant brought on a new series of fears and anxiety that I hadn't completely counted on. I began spotting early on, and even though I knew that to be normal, I found myself calling the nurse frequently to hear her tell me what I already knew. I was normal. I guess I just hadn't felt *normal* in so many years, it was hard to let go of the trepidation.

Tuesday, September 6, 2005
The Tiniest Flicker of Hope

We just got back from the hospital and I'm somewhere between incredibly overjoyed, breathing a sigh of relief, and completely exhausted.

During my grocery shopping today, I started to get some really intense pains. They were very sharp and lasted longer than any of the cramping or pinching I have had over the last week. On my way home I started to feel nervous and started thinking that a trip to the hospital was in order. Something inside me kept telling me this wasn't normal.

On the way there, the pains got worse and I thought for

certain this must be what a miscarriage felt like. Mike went as fast as he could and tried to tell me that everything was going to be fine, but I could tell that he, too, felt the worst was coming.

When we got there, the triage nurse took us right in. She started asking questions and I felt like I was numb to everything. That's when it all started to go further down hill. She told a ridiculous story about a friend of hers who went through IVF six times and never got pregnant, but then got pregnant on her own only to miscarry. She talked about how IVF patients are at a greater risk for miscarriage. I was appalled, but couldn't get myself mad enough to yell **"SHUT UP!"** at her. There was no bright side to this pointless story, only that, she explained, "sometimes a body isn't meant to carry a baby."

The doctor we saw wasn't much better. He was condescending and rude to us. Ultimately though, it didn't matter what his bedside manner was as long as I knew what was going on with me. I ignored his trite comments about this being normal and that I wasn't making the situation better by "carrying on". Too many times in the past I felt like the failed cycles were my fault. Here I was, listening to this moment be my fault as well.

We were sent to the ultrasound room where another doctor did a scan of my stomach. We got to see the gestational sac and the yolk sac, all in the right place. That was a huge relief. I was terrified that we were going to be headed for an ectopic pregnancy, so knowing that the baby was in the right place made me feel so much better. But there was no visible heartbeat and that made me nervous all over again.

The ultrasound guy decided to do a vaginal ultrasound, but still we couldn't see a heartbeat. I knew it was early, but I was flooded with so many terrifying emotions and overwhelmed by ideas of what could be wrong. I had researched all of this and felt an oppressive sense of doom. I held Mike's hand and I watched him stare intently at the screen. The ultrasonographer called in another doctor to look and I felt myself holding my breath.

107

Then suddenly, there it was, the tiniest of tiny little flickers. It was this little flick of light that went from bright white to faded gray and back to bright white again. I could have looked at it all day long. AMAZING! The baby is measuring at 5w2d, but even though it's a little bit behind, I was so elated that it was in the right place and doing the right things.

He continued to look around and explained to us that there was a "boatload" of very large cysts on my ovaries and that was most likely what was causing the pains. He said they would go away eventually, but that the spotting was the larger reason for concern and I really needed to watch out for that.

My blood test came back fine. I'm at 11,237 for the HCG level, which is right where it should be.

So, all signs indicate that the baby and I are okay, and that there is no reason for me to worry about the pains I've been having. Just knowing they aren't related to the health of this baby makes me feel better about them, and I know I can handle any of the spotting and pains for as long as I have to.

And now our little one even has a name... FLICKER!

As the weeks passed, Mike and I started to leave the conversations of infertility behind. In place, we talked about normal things... well almost. Normal people might discuss how much time I could spend with the baby before going back to work. We had this discussion, but it was jaded by the wound of infertility. Not only was there no money to take time off, but we were in debt and that was something that needed to be handled before any time off could be considered. We talked about furniture for the nursery, but we weren't flipping through catalogs with any sense of realistic possibility. We were thinking about which of our friends we could borrow which items from. Infertility had taken a toll, but it was a toll well worth paying for the life that I was carrying.

Pregnant. It was a word I repeated to myself over and over. I loved that word. Pregnant. What a wonderful experience. I didn't have the symptoms of other pregnant women, but that was normal for women in my family. I had leg cramps and extreme thirst. That was about it. I wasn't exhausted. In fact, I was an insomniac for the first month. I would wake up in the middle of the night and stay awake writing in my journal. It didn't bother me that I couldn't sleep. In fact, during the early morning hours when it was just Flicker and me wrapped in a blanket on the couch together, I was more grateful than during the hours when students, friends and family would take my mind away from the little life my body was nourishing.

Wednesday, September 14, 2005
Just You and Me Kid

3:14 a.m. As I type this, you are just a little bundle of cells snuggled into my tummy. I can hardly believe that this is real. Looking at the time, this may very well be a dream, but the constant pinching I've done to my arm proves otherwise.

You don't know who I am and as far as I can see, you are a flickering blip on an ultrasound screen. I don't know if you are a boy or girl, or what color eyes you will have. You don't know what a true miracle you are, nor do you realize how much has been sacrificed for your existence. I don't know if you'll inherit my fiery personality (you and I will call it "passion" and a "zest for life") or your father's natural sense of calm. You don't know that you have a puppy and two cats, or that you have a bedroom that was imagined for you long ago.

There are a lot of uncertainties for all of us, and a lot of decision still to be made. But one thing I am acutely certain of is how deeply you are loved and how desperately you are wanted.

109

You are an amazing little life and in the moment when I learned of you, I felt the years of struggle and pain melt away. You already have an influence over me that I didn't expect. There is nothing I wouldn't repeat to have you here now. In this moment, I have a future I once took for granted, and yet it is because of what it took to bring you here that I treasure you all the more.

You cannot possibly comprehend the power you have. You must have struggled to be the one embryo to make a home here. That was a miraculous effort. You have strength greater than anyone I know and I admire you beyond definition. How can I be so unspeakably proud of someone I haven't even met yet?

I love this moment. The house is dark and quiet except for the hum of the refrigerator. A glow from the computer is the only real light. I imagine this will be a very different experience come May. Maybe I'll be awake with you in my arms, rocking you to sleep for the fifth time in the night. Maybe I'll be in bed listening to your dad read you a book. But right now, it's just you and me together on the couch. As much as I want to learn all about you in the months and years to come, as excited as I am to see who you are and what you will become, I have to selfishly admit that for now you are a lovely little secret. I couldn't be happier in this single moment.

Life could not have been better. Everything that I hoped life would bring was in front of me wrapped up with a giant bow. Each day brought surprises and moments of elation like nothing I had ever experienced. It was easy to see how days that once seemed to drag on were going to fly by now that I was pregnant. I wanted to live in every second and take time to remember each twinge and tingle. Our life had taken a remarkable turn and I began to scrapbook old journal entries to show our child in later years. I pictured our baby as a teenager and ranting as my students sometimes did in a fit of hormones, "You don't really care about me," or "I wish I was never born," to which I would take out this scrapbook and read with him all of the ways that he was brought to us, and he would be silenced by the awe of how intensely loved and desired he, in fact, was.

Friday, September 23, 2005
8w2d

This morning we officially graduated from the fertility clinic after seeing Flicker one more time. She (today it's a girl) had a great heartbeat of 165bpm and was right around the size that she needed to be. My due date seems to be fluctuating, which gives me a few concerns because it keeps being pushed forward as she is growing. Again I'm told this is typical and finally, I am beginning to believe it. The official due date now is May 2nd.

Now we are officially in the hands of a regular obstetrician. It's so strange to think that we won't be going to a fertility clinic any more and that now we are among the normal couples expecting a baby. Of course, not entirely normal just yet; I still have to take the progesterone for three more weeks and the Estrace for two more weeks, but I'm okay with that because I feel like we have a crutch to fall back on until we are almost in the second trimester.

I'm still feeling great. What's nice is that I am starting to get comfortable with the idea that I might just be one of those people who doesn't experience any symptoms and has a great pregnancy, like my sister. I'm not worried as much that this means something bad is happening or that the baby isn't healthy. I know that symptoms may come soon enough or not at all, but that either way the baby is doing what she should be and so am I. With our baby having a healthy and strong heartbeat, I am finally starting to feel comfortable with our future.

I figured I was on a roll with the heartbeat and graduation, so I called an OB/GYN to check on the blood test results. Everything is fine. The only test that hasn't come back is the cystic fibrosis test, but I have already had that one done with the fertility clinic when we first started, so I'm not concerned about it.

We don't see our new doctor for another few weeks, so until then I'm just going to take it easy and continue to think good thoughts. I'll look at the pictures of Flicker and imagine the life we will have. It's a good life, a great life, and I'm looking forward to every moment of it.

We had seen Flicker four times on ultrasound. I marveled at the pictures and spoke to our baby every moment I could. We still hadn't shared our secret with many people outside of our immediate family because we had heard the stories of miscarriages in the first trimester. But for as many of the hideous stories we heard, we were told as many times that once we saw the heartbeat the chances of a miscarriage were in the low single digit percentages and dropped with each passing day. Essentially, our concerns were more a leftover defense from the years of infertility than a realistic possibility.

We started to let go. As we approached the 10th week and going into the 11th, we began to slowly let more and more people in on the pregnancy. Each time, sharing the news felt like the first time. After so many years of being the source for disappointment and pity, it was cathartic to be a source of excitement. Mike and I began thinking of the baby shower and baby names. I had all but forgotten about the painful injections and the tears that were shed.

We were 11 weeks and 4 days pregnant, and ready to hear the heartbeat we had seen so many times. Another little present in this whole remarkable experience. And unlike other moments, this time it didn't feel like an obstacle to overcome. This time, we knew it as yet another amazing experience on our way to being parents. Soon

112

enough we would not only hear the heartbeat, but we would feel the baby kick, and then we would know the gender. There was no trepidation or fear, only excitement and promise.

And then, when everything had begun to fall into place, at the moment of unimaginable hope and unspeakable excitement, the unfathomable happen. Our baby's perfectly healthy heartbeat ceased to beat.

A word from Mike:

I'll admit I wasn't very concerned when we didn't hear the heartbeat with the Doppler during that 11 week appointment. I believed the doctor's explanation that it could sometimes take up to 12 weeks to hear the heartbeat. I thought Jenna was just being emotional. As far as I was concerned, we had already gone through enough on the infertility journey, so everything was going to work out. Jenna outright begged the doctor to order an ultrasound right away. Our doctor agreed to appease her because we had been through so much already. The appointment was set for a few days later, but Jenna again insisted that it be for the following morning. Her panic felt real enough, but I was still certain that she was just experiencing remnants of past fears. It wasn't until that night that I began to feel differently.

When I first learned that I was going to be a father, I began working on finishing part of the third floor in the attic. The goal was to move my office up there in order to make it quieter at night for the baby when I had to work late. Every night I spent an hour or two working on the room. I remember very distinctly hanging up a piece of molding when all of a sudden a feeling of dread overwhelmed me. The sense of urgency I had to work on the room in the weeks before was immediately gone. I didn't want to let on to Jenna how I was feeling.

The next morning I had requested only a few hours off of work to go on the appointment, convincing myself everything was fine. I even gained some confidence as we entered the doctor's office. The waiting room was decorated very tastefully with elevator music playing quietly in the background. It all provided a sense of hope to me. Jenna went in first, as was their protocol, and I would be invited in once the important measurements were taken. I decided to thumb through a magazine while waiting to be brought to the ultrasound room. Once the door opened in the waiting room, the next 36 hours became an absolute blur.

A nurse called my name and led me towards the room. As she was about to open the door, she told me that Jenna was extremely upset because there was no heartbeat found. I had approximately one second to soak up that information before I walked in to see my wife. I didn't understand what she was saying. The words were in English, but the message didn't make sense. We were just there to reassure Jenna. We were going to see the baby and Jenna was going to feel silly for making such a big deal over this. The nurse's words were incomprehensible.

Jenna was crying and looked extremely weak. I had to be strong for the both of us, so I blocked out the shock and sadness related to the miscarriage in order to comfort her. The doctor came in and went over our options. We could wait hours or days to miscarry naturally at home. We could take a medication to induce the loss, or Jenna could go into surgery and have the baby removed. Within seconds, we had made the decision to go forward with a D&E. Immediately, Jenna stopped crying and turned into a new person, completely rational and businesslike. She began *asking questions about the process of testing the baby for abnormalities and wanted to have it done as soon as possible. Seeing the obvious sense of urgency on her face, our doctor made special arrangements to do the procedure that afternoon.*

The next thing I remember is seeing bloody bandages laying in a bucket near her bed in the recovery room. Jenna was still groggy from the procedure when I took my first second to process it all. There was so much blood. How could these bandages really be from my wife? It was at that point I realized just how much she had gone through and how strong of a person she was. She woke up later and burst into hysterical tears unlike anything I've ever seen before or since. I realized as I looked into her swelled eyes, those blood-soaked wrappings weren't just from my wife; they were from our baby.

Friday, October 14, 2005

2 weeks ago

2 weeks ago I was researching the size of my baby.

2 weeks ago I was looking through baby furniture web sites for cribs and dressers.

2 weeks ago Mike and I were making lists of projects that needed to be done before May.

2 weeks ago that baby's heart stopped, and I didn't even know it.

24 hours ago I had every dream in my life coming true.

24 hours ago I was looking forward to maternity leave and baby showers.

24 hours ago I was a mom to a beautiful, brilliant little baby.

24 hours ago I was about to pick up my latest picture of Flicker.

Today I am recovering from the surgery that ripped that baby away.

Today life bleeds from me.

Today I am 24 hours past sleep and eating, and I don't desire either.

Today seems incredibly far from yesterday and even further away from tomorrow.

Of all the disappointments and losses I'd experienced to that point, never had the depth of heartbreak been so transforming. I had loved our baby so completely. I had envisioned laughing with that child until I was brought to tears and wiping away the tears after breakups and bad grades. I walked with our child to kindergarten and watched our young adult walk the stage to receive a high school diploma. I experienced first dates and first loves. In the weeks that followed the loss of our baby, someone said to me, "Thank goodness you weren't further along." How could that person possibly know that I had lived a lifetime in those 11 weeks and 4 days?

Monday, October 17, 2005

Falling Off an Orbiting World

People still laugh. They still talk about their inane disappointments and frustrations. They forward emails to me with jokes that probably weren't funny before and definitely aren't funny now. The world keeps turning while my life has come to an abrupt halt.

Nothing. I'm searching for something to care about; something to reignite that passion I had for my job, my home, my family. Nothing. I feel myself walking through my day wasting time until I can sit on the couch and stare through the television. My consciousness fades away and I find myself suddenly sitting at my desk, or walking in the hall and not knowing how I got there.

I went to the bathroom at school and staring at me is a poster that read, "Life is Good" and I think, "For who?" and a voice whispers shyly back, "For you Jenna. Life is still good for you". Even my own sub-conscious can't humor me.

I look in a mirror and think, "I look so much better than I feel." And that makes me angry, because I want the world to see me as the vacant shell that I feel I am. I want them all to notice and say something trite to me like, "It will happen when it's meant to be" or "Everything happens for a reason." Just one person needs to say this so I can get angry and explode in a rant of all the emotions I have of bitterness and rage. But they stay away.

My stomach growls. I hate that I'm hungry. My own body is rejecting my desire to shut down completely. Can't it do just one thing right for me?

Did anyone notice that I fell off the earth four days ago? I did. I am hanging on by my fingernails and all I need to do is let myself go. It would be so much easier to just let go of everything. But where did this fighter come from? It's Hope. She was so quiet and I thought she was my weakness all those years and cycles ago.

Yet here she is, stronger than any other part of me. Her grip is intense and she isn't going to let me go.

Perhaps it was the years of infertility that had made me stronger; strong enough to continue living each day, continue going to work, and putting a smile on for the kids I taught, the kids who were a constant reminder of what I had lost only days earlier.

I don't believe it was time that healed this wound. I believe it was the love I had for Mike and the gratitude I had for a life I didn't always feel that I deserved. I didn't want to lose the only parts of that life that were solid and safe, even though the rest of me felt intensely fragile.

There was more of that life to come. I had been pregnant. That was more than a lot of women get, and I knew it was something to be thankful for. I had experienced a miracle even for too brief a time.

Thursday, October 20, 2005

No Place for Pity

Was it Arthur Ashe who said something about not asking, "Why me" in the face of disappointment or tragedy? I am beginning to understand that.

When the clock in my classroom struck 9:45 a.m., I was paralyzed at my desk. I stared at the clock until the minute had passed as if that one minute was the last minute of my life and I was seeing it all flash before my eyes. It's been exactly one week since I lost our baby.

The minute passed as they all tend to do, and I was still there. I knew the week was over and I was still standing, still alive. And even though I can so easily relive the moments of my life during that brief time in the dark room surrounded by ultrasound equipment, the fact is, it is now the past.

And also I know that I cannot leave room for self-indulgent pity. My life is so full of wonderful people, proven 10-fold by the support I've had this week, that to do anything beyond being thankful for those things is just selfish. Was I saying, "Why me?" when I was blessed that the IVF had worked? Was I looking for a reason when I had the support of my parents, both financially and emotionally, as we went through these processes? Did I once question why I was able to walk down the aisle and meet Mike crying at our wedding? Of course not. I have experienced amazing things in my life and phenomenal things are still to come.

If it is true that nothing is free in this life, then that would explain a lot of what's going on and it gives me hope for what is ahead. I look back at how some of the major experiences in my life have unfolded and it seems that they have usually come on the heels of some kind of tragedy or trying time.

I look at my parents and they love each other so much. I have such an appreciation for that only because of what I saw them endure in my early childhood. Like many relationships, theirs wasn't always easy and they certainly had their share of arguments and darker times. Had I not had that history or seen those challenging times, I don't think I would see how important a relationship is or admire theirs as I do today.

I have always had financial battles to face. I was one of those people who got sucked into credit card debt from the first application that bore my name. Before graduating college, I had racked up tens of thousands of dollars of debt, so I know how emotionally draining money problems can be. Because I had to face that challenge and overcome it, I am more careful with my money today, and I know that I have to save money for my children and retirement. The value of a dollar is greater when you know what it's like to not have a single one to your name.

I was not a great student in school. I know what it feels like to panic on a math test and feel like a failure. I understand how it feels to want to hide from a teacher's questions and not want to be called on or even have a teacher remembered. Because of my own experiences of feeling inadequate, I am now a teacher who thrives when faced with those students who are like me and I can help them to feel successful and express themselves.

And there is so much more... My husband, home, my pets, my family, my friends... they are all a part of a life that I have created. And this life all comes from learning lessons and making sacrifices that at the time seemed insurmountable; problems that I didn't think I would be able to overcome and moments where I felt that I was being punished for bad karma or poor choices.

And this, losing Flicker, seems insurmountable. It has only been nine days since our baby was taken from me and there are times that I get angry and sad at this loss. Yet at the same time, I understand that I'm just learning a lesson or paying a price in advance for something that I will find myself treasuring in the years to come.

Does this mean everything happens for a reason? I'm not sure about that. Certainly there are other ways to learn lessons in life. Not everyone has to endure difficult times to be happy. Some people are "charmed" and seem to just have life handed to them. I'm still working on not being jealous or bitter about that. But at the least, I know that I am still standing after things that would crush a different person.

No, there is no room for pity here. There is room for gratitude and awe for the parts of my life that have passed and the moments still to come. There is no room for pity here.

But for every moment of stunning clarity, would come a more lasting moment of emotional torture. A reality of the life I had lost inside me would throw me back into defeat. I was on a seesaw of fantastic gratitude and unspeakable heartbreak. I was sitting on both sides at the same time. What pushed me from one side to the next was anyone's guess. It might be a commercial for diapers, or a song on the radio, or a moment of quiet when there was nothing to distract me from my truth. In those moments, there was no consolation or peace for my internal turmoil, only a deep sadness unlike any other I had imagined. It was a sadness that pervaded every cell of my being and an emptiness that ran through my veins and into my heart, which seemed as natural as the blood that carried it there.

Wednesday, November 2, 2005

CONGRATULATIONS, it was a boy

The doctor called with the results of the chromosomal testing on the "product of conception".

Everything was normal. It was a healthy male.

A What?

A male.

I had a boy?

It was a healthy boy. All chromosomes in the right place.

I had a son.

Yes, you did.

Breathless. In a split second I
am both elated and devastated.
I shouldn't know this for a few more weeks.

Reality. I know this because he is no longer alive.
I didn't *have* a miscarriage.
I *had* a son.
A baby boy. Our first child. Our first son.

Time would pass, and as time tends to do, the strength and hope for a future came back to both Mike and I. We had faced our greatest fear and while we were worn and scraped, we were still standing. More importantly, we were standing side by side. Our relationship had been pushed to yet another place where it could have weakened a lesser couple. I saw Mike differently after the loss of our son. He was a different man, more serious, focused and stronger than he had been before. He had matured in the last few months and though I didn't think I could have loved him more, I truly did. There we were, together and firm in our commitment to each other and the family we were certain we would have.

Over the course of the next few months we would go through a battery of rigorous testing to attempt to determine the cause of our miscarriage. In addition to those processes, I was haunted with the continued positive pregnancy test. It seems strange, doesn't it? I had worked so hard for this pregnancy and in the end, the baby clung to me well after his heart stopped beating. The hormones that rushed through my bloodstream continued to show that I was pregnant for well over a month after the loss. I would go in for a blood test every few days and then every week or two. Each time, the nurse would tell me it was still reading pregnant. How ironic, that we had come so far to be pregnant and there we were hoping for a negative result.

We felt confident that if I could get pregnant once, I could get pregnant again. We were more determined to stay the course than ever. The time between cycles allowed me to regain some of my strength back that had been lost during the exhaustion of the miscarriage. I hadn't realized how tired I was emotionally and physically until the last pregnancy test over Thanksgiving weekend finally returned negative. It was only then that I was able to mourn the loss the way I needed to.

Thursday, November 24, 2005

Giving Thanks

This is a tough one. I'm almost ready to head out the door and travel to Thanksgiving dinner where I will have the good fortune of surrounding myself with family and amongst them, children. Once again I will feel another year of feeling left out. No one will make me feel that way, in fact no one will mention anything about the obvious fact that Mike and I don't have any children. I used to be grateful that we had a family and friends where no one put pressure on us to have kids. I enjoyed the privacy we were afforded. It's odd though. It doesn't feel like privacy anymore. Lately, it feels more like avoidance. Like it's obvious we don't have kids. We've been together for nine years and married for three, and we don't have a baby. I think everyone has come to realize this isn't a choice for us. We are the elephant in the room, but as long as they can claim to respect our privacy, it can't be called avoidance. Hmmm... *Don't make them the bad guys, Jenna. You are just looking for someone to take the brunt of the loose cannon of emotions right now.*

I have been trying to be optimistic and every once in a while I have these moments where I get genuinely excited about the holidays coming. I turn on the radio and listen to Christmas music, and try to think about how lucky I am to have everything and everyone that I do. I look around the house and think about decorating and wrapping presents.

But this is one of those moments where I am not terribly convincing.

The television is filled with commercials where children are opening toys and news of miracle births from impossible accidents where the mother and baby never should have survived. The stores have pregnant women and mothers pushing around their carriages with babies inside. They anger me. How dare they act so put off by the inconvenience of their own children? I remember buying this house and envisioning a family around a Christmas tree.

I can't help but think about how different this holiday would have been if I still had our baby. Today would be the first day I would see my family since my mom would have called to let them all know the good news. I would be showing up at dinner with ultrasound pictures and stories of how lucky we are to have this little one. People would be so amazed to hear the war stories of IVF, and the blessing might even be focused on welcoming our baby next May.

I would be feeling him move by now, but still not know whether it was a boy or girl. I'd be sharing ideas of baby names, all the while knowing that there was really only one name if it was a boy and a few if it was a girl. What would I be wearing by now? How would I be feeling? We'd be laughing about how this is the last holiday where Mike and I will get presents because they'd all be for the baby next year.

Instead our son isn't here, and no one at dinner will even know he existed, because we lost him three days shy of telling the world. I can't stop myself from going down that road of "what if" and hating the fact that I have a size two pair of pants on and no sign of anything different in the future. I miss him. I miss the idea of him and the reality of him. I miss the way I felt when I had a little secret that no one else knew, and I miss the experience of sharing that secret with those closest to me. I miss who Mike was when he was going to be a father, and I miss who I was when I was finally able to give him that. I've lost something more profound than I could have imagined, and no matter what the future holds, I will never have another first son.

Nonetheless, I refuse to sit at the table today and silently say, "Thanks for Nothing"... I know how fortunate I am. I am married to a truly amazing man and I have parents who would, and have, gone to the end of the earth for me, both with material goods and emotionally. These things I do not take lightly. No matter how lost and lonely I feel, I am reminded each day that we have so much more to be thankful for and there has to be more ahead for us. But, as I sit here with my coat on, ready to leave, I just don't know what that is.

By the time we had reached the third round of IVF, we had officially spent every dime in our savings, not to mention the generous contributions of my parents. We were in debt and feeling the gravity of reality. Rationally, we knew our chances were the same as they were during the first round, but emotionally and financially, we were attached to this process, for better or worse. There was no longer an "adoption option" as the catch phrase boasted. We did research adoption as we had decided, and when we learned that it could cost around $30,000, that kind of debt was impossible to amass. Even prior to our issues of infertility, adoption at this cost would have been difficult to swallow, but at the place we were in, $30,000 was out of the question. Of course we could probably find a less expensive agency and there might be a tax credit we could employ, but still, this figure was astounding. Another round of IVF at $10,000 seemed daunting, but at that point we were in a situation that was being dictated by a home equity loan, and the process which required the least debt possible was the only reasonable course.

In December of that year, I underwent my second

hysteroscopy. The first one had been just prior to the IVF which resulted in the pregnancy. This one was important to ensure that no damage had been done during the D&E procedure following the miscarriage. Specifically, there was a concern about scar tissue from the procedure that might prevent further pregnancy. During the surgery, the doctor removed "product of conception." There were remnants of the fetus still attached to the uterus. This realization was difficult to swallow. On the one hand, I felt like our baby had been once and for all scrapped from me and effectively erased from existence. On the other hand, I was in dire need of a fresh start and ready to put the past behind me.

As we prepared for the next IVF, I felt confident that it would work. I believed wholeheartedly that we had found the magic potion, the right mix of medications to create the eggs and embryos that we needed. I was especially comfortable knowing that the cycle that resulted in our son was under the worst circumstances. We had lost all of the embryos except for him, proving that "it only takes one." I couldn't have had a more positive attitude or greater hope for the following cycle.

We took the gamble again in the beginning of the next year. Once again, it was the same rigorous routine of medications and the same excitement for another possible pregnancy. But at the end of the seven week stretch of birth control, stimulation, retrieval, transfer and pregnancy test, we lost. Nothing had gone wrong. The cycle was as it should have been. I was eating well, getting a lot of sleep, meditating and concentrating all of my focus on the future. I didn't feel any pressure of stress, and had more faith and confidence than ever before. The embryos were of "textbook" quality. Even the endometrial lining, which had caused me such concern in the past, seemed to be right where it should be. There was no obvious reason for this to fail. But it had. Like so many other times, it wasn't just a cycle that failed, it was me who was the weak link.

I remember a time after this third IVF cycle when I began to question this path. I had never wavered before. Even after the miscarriage, I did not feel that God had given me this calling to be a mother senselessly. If anything, I felt more impassioned and more focused for what I believed I was to do. But this failure, perhaps because of that intense conviction, affected my trust in that purpose. Why would I be given such an amazing gift of love for children and be unable to apply it to my husband and myself? It was the first time that my faith was shaken. I had been let down and crushed by the news of a failed cycle on numerous occasions prior to this, but the pain of the failure had never gone to the deepest part of my soul the way this one had.

Tuesday, February 21, 2006
What Now?

Mike is having a tougher time with this than any of the previous cycles. He slept for nearly two days straight this weekend and even last night went to bed around 8:00. Unheard of! He emailed me from work yesterday saying that he was "having a hard time blending in" and "just wanted to be left alone." This is the first time he's cracked a bit on being able to be strong for me when we are given the bad news. I didn't know what to do for him. He's the sweetest guy in the world, and although he may not look it overtly, he is immensely strong at heart and his will is admirable. It is because of me that he is hurting right now. I know we are in it together, but the reality of the situation is that it is MY body that isn't working here and while Mike would NEVER blame me, I certainly do.

I love that man more than I can write in words. He has literally saved my life when I was on the brink of self consuming depression. He has been strength for me when mine was all but extinct. Mike has been my conscience, my confidence and my will at times when I was lacking in all of those things. It may be because of his belief in me and this relationship that I now feel so worthless. I can't give him a child. With anyone else he would have a baseball team of kids. With me he gives and gives, and I cannot return the most basic human function even with an army of physicians behind me.

I worry about what we will be like at the end. When everything has fallen into place, whether through IVF, adoption or childless, what will Mike and I be like? Will we still be the same people we've known for so many years? Will we love each other more for these trials? I have a vision in my head that we are stronger with each passing cycle, and yet, right now, as I type these words, with my husband sleeping upstairs for the 4th early night in a row, I feel weaker than ever before.

Guilt, so much guilt. I am exhausted of the constant ache in my heart. Something stronger than me keeps me going on this path when my entire being wants to be angry and give up. I have faith that whatever that is, it will get me through these times. But that faith is slowly ebbing. Being a mom was never an option in my soul. It was not a choice I made. It was something I thought I was meant to be; like a predestined plan from a higher power. It felt that strong in my heart. Now, it feels like a cruel joke of which I am the butt.

I feel like things are falling apart. How did we get to this place? How has so much time passed since the days of taking my temperature and eating food to gain weight? And all of this for nothing. There must be something we are missing. I had every bit of faith in this cycle. Why would we be given the pregnancy earlier if we were supposed to give in and move on? I feel like this is a struggle every day, and for what? For something that maybe I wasn't meant to have?

I don't know what to do if I'm not meant to be anyone's mom; the thought has never been more than a fleeting one... a "what if... but I won't think of that now" kind of thought. Yet here I am, and every day that passes I get closer and closer to a reality and a conversation that I know will need to happen.

I wish I could forward time and see if I would have children. I just need to know... not the when, but just yes or no. That way I can stop all this commotion in my head and not feel so damn crazy all the time. Each time we get into a new protocol it seems to monopolize my life until I can feel every twinge and every ache... until I'm making up the twinges and aches just to will myself to move forward.

I'm trying to be proactive and think ahead. It's getting harder and harder to bounce back into things after a disappointment. I am so afraid that one day there won't be any bouncing. One day it will be more difficult to start a cycle than to end one. At some point the pain of going through it again will be worse than that of learning it didn't work. I can hear that time knocking, but I'm not answering, yet.

Chapter 7

*Scraping the Bottom of the
Infertility Barrel*

Ifeel it would be unfair to neglect the fact that a significant number of infertility patients will never have to experience the repeated failures that Mike and I did. Technology is constantly advancing. IVF and its related techniques can produce wonders. Those miracle babies are everywhere. They are the children of celebrities and they walk among us normal folks, too. The population will only increase over the next few generations. If you are just beginning your infertility journey, please don't let my experiences scare you. Chances are very good that, depending on your reason for needing treatments, you will have a biological child. But for some of us, the veterans of infertility, the quest becomes a much longer one.

We had eight embryos cryogenically preserved from the first and third IVF. Cycling with those was a much less expensive procedure and didn't require the high doses of medications or the painful egg retrieval, since the embryos already existed. That was the good news. The bad news was that the success rates rivaled those of the IUI days. Still there seemed to be a lot of research showing that some women respond better because they aren't on as many meds. It was worth a shot (or a few dozen if I'm being literal).

To prepare for the Frozen Embryo Transfer (FET), Mike and I decided that I should work with an acupuncturist for a few months. Since that seemed to be the one thing that differentiated the positive cycle from the others, it was well worth the three-month commitment that was required to prepare my body. At the tune of $85 per week, I was taking herbal concoctions three times a day and getting stuck with needles once each week. In addition, the suggestion was made to implement an all organic diet. We did. It nearly doubled our grocery bill to $160 per week, but I felt great. By the time we were ready to cycle, I felt physically and emotionally stronger than I had felt since the pregnancy and even prior to. I was confident that this was going to make the difference.

Once again, we began the shots of Lupron to suppress my system from ovulating. I wasn't on the other medications to stimulate egg production, and I have to say that felt 100% better. Without the side effects from the high dose meds, I was operating like my normal self on a regular basis. I didn't know if it was the addition of acupuncture or the lack of meds, or even just that we had done this so many times, but the cycle went by with the snap of a finger. Suddenly, we were at the embryo transfer and watching the miracle of our future on the screen before our eyes.

Sadly, it wasn't the miracle we had prayed for. The embryos were deemed "marginal" upon thawing. Even with three transferred, we were left with another devastating failure.

And this failure would later be followed by a second FET failure the following summer.

If this is sounding like the same sad song stuck on repeat, it felt that way, too. The years of trying to conceive a baby were exhausting. We had made a deal in the very beginning that we were a team, and we would stick together until *both* of us were ready to put an end to the whole thing. At this point, I was ready. We had already begun looking into adoption, and had been given a generous offer from a friend to be a surrogate for us. I wanted off the ride. Even though it was my body that was taking the brunt of the physical torment, Mike's heart was as invested in the successes and failures as mine. Deal or no deal, I knew Mike would have conceded to ending the processes, but I was not about to make that decision for both of us. I knew he had to come to a place of acceptance in his own way and at his own time.

We went to see another specialist with a different approach who convinced us that things would be different with their protocol. We were easily persuaded; to say "convinced" is probably not the most accurate description. When you want to believe something badly enough, there is no need to sell an idea. It didn't take more than, "You're only 31 years old" and "We've had a remarkable success rate with people in your situation." We were 100% sold on another round of treatment.

Another battery of testing would reveal that neither Mike nor I carried any specific genetic marker that could explain our past failures. A third hysteroscopy was performed and once again, everything came up clean and structurally sound. We ordered our medications and promptly signed ourselves up for our 4th round trip through IVF hell and back. Another generous contribution from my parents' retirement savings would help fund another fresh cycle. Another round of injections, side effects, and emotional turmoil resulted in another cycle of bitter disappointment. Another enormous dose of guilt with a chaser of shame was mine to swallow.

It couldn't simply be amenorrhea that was causing the problem. Fifteen embryos of amazing quality have been transferred throughout the procedures. Amenorrhea had nothing to do with that. It wasn't a lack of positive thinking or stress. Even in the very end, I was able to find humor in the technology and I was as optimistic as possible that "it only takes one." My doctor was certain that my uterus was structurally sound. It was something else that we couldn't determine. The bottom line was that I just couldn't get pregnant and stay that way. Next to eating and sleeping, I couldn't perform the very function of human existence: to procreate.

There is a shame in infertility that is difficult to express. People's immediate reaction is to say something like, "No, there's no reason to feel ashamed." They want to follow this up with an anecdote or an antidote. This, yet another well-intentioned comment, is incredibly dismissive. When I hear these words, they immediately translate themselves into, "Infertility is not that big of a deal." The fact is, this isn't a stylish disease. It's not en vogue to be a reproductive failure, the way it is for celebrities to bounce in and out of drug rehab like it's a vacation resort. People who fight other diseases are hailed as heroes; strong, courageous and determined. They write books on their recovery and people wonder how they had the strength to keep going when so many odds were against them.

I felt a quiet shame in that I didn't feel courageous or strong. I felt weak and useless. I hadn't been given the option of having biological kids or not. I never made the choice not to reproduce. I wasn't one of those people who decided to focus on my career or travel with my spouse. I didn't have lofty goals of dedicating my life to world peace. What I wanted was simple, I thought. I wanted a family and what didn't seem like too much to ask for was more than I could have. In some ways, I began to feel that perhaps it was more than I deserved.

I also felt selfish. The failures had brought repeated pain to not only my husband and me, but to our families. My parents specifically had helped to financially support every cycle that we couldn't. They had told us that they would do whatever they could to help, and we took full advantage of that. Not only were they emotionally invested in our family building, but they had sacrificed some of their retirement savings as well. Sometimes, I thought it would be easier to give up on our unborn children than to cause these people who actually existed even more pain.

Chapter 8

The Devolution of the Infertile

I nfertility changes a person. Whether I ever get pregnant again or whether I have a dozen kids, infertility will be something that will be a part of my life long after the pain and anxiety of cycling fades. Often I feel unrecognizable from the person I once knew. Every aspect of who I am has been altered by the veil of infertility.

This disease doesn't scar the heart, it bruises the soul. A scar might be permanent in appearance, but is easily forgotten. The wound that caused it scabs over and flakes off. The remaining tissue can be covered up with makeup and causes no lasting pain. Some people even brag about their battle scars. But the bruise of infertility is far deeper than a surface scar. It is the bruise you receive in the place that is constantly being grazed. Just when you think you have let go of the pain, you bump it again and it immediately turns a deep purple. This bruise doesn't disappear. Deep below the surface the composition of my being has been transformed by it. Long after a cycle is over, this disease changes the way I think, talk and act. Infertility isn't simply disappointment, it is all but devastating.

Friday, February 24, 2006
Where Did I Go So Long Ago?

I don't know what to say. It's been such a hard week. I feel like a bomb has exploded and taken every dream I've had. I wish it had taken me. But instead I get to stay here and live this fragmented and disfigured life in the shadow of what I once loved. I get to live life looking at other people hold my dreams frivolously in their hands, without knowing how easily they could have come to not having them either.

I'm sad and scared, and so angry at myself for not being strong enough to have friends who have happy lives and deal with this, too. I've prided myself for being courageous and strong, and I hate that these years have changed me so much from the person they've known. And with that comes more guilt.

These people were once my friends. They were the people who were traveling on the same track as Mike and I, and now things are so painfully different. I can't sit in a room with them without feeling like the outsider. They play with their kids on the floor and talk about all the new things their babies are doing. They can go to anyone's home and have enough toys to keep their children occupied for hours. Not at our house. Here they play with the dog toys.

I sit on the outside of conversations and smile when I can, but I have nothing to offer. Their lives are so distant from mine. Could I pretend to understand what they are interested in? Only to the degree that they can understand what I'm going through. It's essentially a false friendship, void of what we shared years and decades ago. But I keep pretending. I keep going to these events;

birthday parties, barbeques, and baptisms. I pray for a day when I will be able to be the friend I once was instead of the fifth wheel I feel I constantly am.

This is really starting to eat away at me from the inside. In so many ways I feel like a shell of who I once was. I don't know how to smile anymore. I try, but tears come down instead. For no reason, or maybe for every reason, I just don't know anymore. I don't remember the last time I genuinely laughed and meant it.

The facade I put up everyday is crumbling. The tougher I try to be, the weaker I feel. The nurse at my doctor's office called me today out of the blue. She was worried about me; said when she last saw me I looked sad and pained, and that I can't keep holding it all in; that I laughed too much for it to be sincere. I cried. She's right. I'm scared. My mind knows the secret that we are nearing the end and my heart is fighting it. My soul is caught in the middle.My heart is breaking. Maybe it's already broken. I can't feel it anymore.

So who am I now? Am I better for this experience? Is my relationship with my husband stronger for the pain and heartache? Romantically, I want to say unequivocally, "YES!" The truth is, we are financially fractured, and physically, my body is exhausted. The constant unpredictability of side effects from the medications has wreaked havoc on my body coming in the form of constant fatigue, nausea, and mood swings. Emotionally, I am certainly more fragile than I'd like. I find myself sensitive to the most well-intentioned comments, and the cry of a baby can send me into a tailspin from which it can take hours to recover.

Mike and I have experienced the deaths of a half dozen family and friends, eight moves to five different towns, a business together, eight employment changes and four animals. We've faced more life-changing decisions than many people at our stage in life. With each new experience we looked to each other for strength and confidence to do what we felt was right. I would say we were even a bit cocky about the fortitude of our relationship by the time we got married. But infertility was an entirely new deck of cards. It didn't just change me, or Mike, it changed us.

Wednesday, August 30, 2006
What Doesn't Kill You, Might Just Kill You Eventually

When we got our first glimpse that we would have to work to conceive child, I would surf through chat rooms and listen to women tell agonizing stories about whether they should pursue the possibilities of artificial insemination or in vitro fertilization. Those were such foreign ideas to me. To be honest, I didn't even know there was a difference. At that point, I was so new to the whole thing that I couldn't imagine that using a thermometer would be able to get anyone pregnant. Months later, after taking my first round of Clomid, I was shocked to find myself even considering other means of high tech conception. Now here I am, after two failed rounds of IUI, three fresh IVF cycles and two FETs, and our thoughts and daily conversations are involving even more remote possibilities for conception.

Whatever happened to "How was your day?" Now our first questions to each other are about whether I've called the doctor, or researched alternative medicines, or whether Mike has thought any further about the other ways we can finance adoption or surrogacy. I can easily see how this journey to parenthood can takes its toll on a relationship.

I used to think that if something like trying to conceive could hurt a marriage, then that is probably a sign that the relationship shouldn't be bringing children into the world; that it wasn't meant to last to begin with. That was when I thought we were invincible. That was when I would flaunt around the fact that Mike and I had been through so much and we were so strong together. Now, as I think back on the nights of tears, anger, disappointment and frustration, I wonder how anyone manages to get through this in one piece.

I am immensely grateful that Mike and I are on the same page with this, but it wasn't always that way. I remember the arguments and frustrations too well. Like all of the negative pregnancy tests, these moments have left their marks. Where I was anxious to get on with medical treatments, and sink us into debt if it meant moving forward, Mike was always more rational and logical. It angered me that he could reduce my pain to a formula on an Excel spreadsheet. In the midst of my emotional battles, I often misunderstood his level-headedness for ambivalence. We both wanted to be parents and we both felt that we need to continue aggressively pursuing a plan. We just didn't always agree on which plan, and sometimes in the middle of the arguments we forgot the bigger picture and disagreements on the details became personal attacks. It was in the heat of battle that I felt so tired and beaten. At those times, I understood the chat rooms I've lurked in where women, who I used to think were so pathetic, discuss their concerns that their spouses aren't on the same page as they are. I wonder how an experience like this could ever make a couple stronger. I wonder how the trials of decision-making and compromise could do anything but push people away.

People keep telling me that maybe we won't have a family the traditional way, but we WOULD have a family. I think this is supposed to be a pep talk. I'm about three years past the pep talk stage. I laugh. I know they mean well, but who said anything about a traditional family? We gave up on that notion years ago when I took my first pill and gave myself the first of literally hundreds upon hundreds of injections, and wrote our first of many checks for what has amounted to approximately $60,000, depleting every resource we have and even some resources we didn't know we had. Traditional family? HA! I just want a family that includes more than the furry herd of Cleo, Jordan and Fenway.

But there is a future. This I know. We are not without hope for that. We are never down for long and we always find a way to keep going. There is an end to this somewhere, or else I wouldn't have this aching drive that persists in my soul to parent. There isn't always an immediate plan, maybe not today, but certainly by tomorrow... or at least the day after that!

This week we talked about selling the house. *It's just a house,* I tell myself. *It's an empty space craving a family that we can't provide it.* But in the same breath my sentimental side remembers driving around the neighborhood for the first time, hanging out of windows to paint it, and the housewarming barbeque that has become a yearly tradition. What once felt like a home, now reminds us of an open wound. We sit in a "family room" and together, we are the only family we have. We need money for adoption or surrogacy, or donor eggs, and ironically, it will need to come from the structure in which we wanted to raise those children. We had a realtor look at the house to see what we can get for it. The answer was dismal. The market just isn't in our favor, then again, what is?

So instead, tonight we are selling both of our cars. A decision and a compromise. We are stronger than our cars and our foundation is more solid than any house we live in.

Perhaps one of the greatest tragedies in all of this is the effect it has had on our friendships. Friendships that stemmed from a common path and common goals, suddenly became foreign. There was no way for someone who has children to understand the depth of sadness that Mike and I feel each day for our countless losses. For them, having children was a choice they made one day and probably thought very little of the process by which their family would be created. They can't possibly understand how all encompassing this journey is, because for them it was natural and private. Each month they tried for their babies that ended in a normal period, they felt disappointment, and maybe they even shed a tear of concern, but they cannot conceive of the humiliation brought about by the constant invasion of privacy and prodding questions in regards to our most intimate habits as husband and wife.

Conversations that were once easy and fluid are pained and awkward between our friends and us. The experiences where we are all together, like in our college years, happen when there is a child's birthday, a baby shower, or a baptism. These are no places for the infertile. But I tried. I tried because I cared deeply for these friends. I treasured the history we shared and wanted to create memories for the future. It was the present that was the problem and the more I tried to fix it, the worse it became.

Sunday, January 7, 2007

Mirror, Mirror on the Wall

Who's the worst friend of them all?

I've done this before. I thought I was prepared. I had practiced a million different conversations in my head and some I even practiced out loud. I left the house and was ready for an assortment of situations. I felt confident that I could go to our nephew's third birthday without having a repeat of last year's nightmare where I cried through the hours until Mike took me home. But this past Saturday, all of the hopes for new memories were pretty much shattered. I'm entering a new phase of emotions. This one is ugly and downright nasty. I worry that this one is here to stay.

It was Jack's birthday and as much as I love him, this was the last place I wanted to be. We walked in the house and it was a stereotypical three-year-old's birthday party; balloons, hats, signs, and twenty other toddlers running all over the place. There was screaming, laughing, crying... the whole bit. If I didn't realize that I didn't fit in, it was painfully obvious when it was clear that I was the only woman in the room who didn't have a child appendage strapped to my leg or arm. Every mock conversation I had in the mirror while getting ready was gone. I couldn't remember anything, not even my preplanned excuses to leave the room.

Mike said he wouldn't leave my side. Usually I get stuck with the women and children in the living room while he gets to drink beers with the boys. He stayed true to his word and we spent some time talking to my parents. I started to feel more at ease. I blocked out the kids on the floor and their mothers laughing and joking about their newest acquired abilities. I promised myself that I would talk to them later, but I had to get my bearings first. I was doing okay. I was doing more than okay. I'd say I was pretty damn impressive. I did not break into tears even when surrounded by a friend who was pregnant with her second baby and my sister, happily pregnant with twins. Any infertile would appreciate how difficult that must have been.

But then it happened. At a moment I was least prepared for. My sister came up to me just as another friend walked in the door with her husband and one and a half-year-old son. She pulled me to the side and whispered, "Jenna, I have to tell you before you find out. She is pregnant again."

It was like a brick had been thrown across the room and hit me directly in my heart. Bitter numbness in my fingers and toes, and all the blood that had left my extremities, rushed to my head. The noises of screaming children, laughter, and adult conversations swirled around my head in a whirlwind. I felt dizzy and suddenly incredibly breathless. Looking back now, I can feel it like it was a second ago. Was this a panic attack? I don't know. I grabbed a bottle of water and went to the second floor, safely out of sight of anyone. I locked myself in the bathroom and cried in a way I hadn't remembered since the loss of our son.

I came out an hour or so later, just as the dining room was filled with dozens of people singing "Happy Birthday." I don't think anyone even noticed I was gone. I am truly grateful for that; the humiliation would have been crushing. Yet, at the same time, the fact that my absence was unrealized speaks volumes as to how totally insignificant I feel.

God, I must have looked like the most depressed person. I sat in a chair while the people around me shared stories of their babies. I looked dead ahead when Mike, who was sitting next to me, held one of the toddlers born a year ago and was now a crawling, spunky little person. I never even glanced at another friend whose baby I had not yet met. And when another friend tried to talk to me about school and non-child related issues while holding her child innocently in her arms, I couldn't even carry on a normal adult conversation.

What a bitch I was. And I knew it. I couldn't even fake it. I couldn't even come close to pretending that I was having fun. I hate myself for that. It's not okay. It's mean and selfish, and I hate that this is who I am. I don't want to be bitter. I don't want to turn every moment into a moment about me and my sadness. It is never my intention, but it is always my impact.

I need to look at myself. This past weekend a rather large mirror was held up to my face. I don't like the person looking back at me. I don't like that I can be happy and have fun, and then within seconds a trigger to the wounds of the past years sends me into a tailspin; each one harder and harder to recover from. I can't be surprised when I don't get invited out to lunches with my girlfriends and their kids, or the picnic at the beach during the summer. I don't even want to be around me, why would they?

No one seemed able to understand the pain I felt just by walking into an event like this. I tried to imagine how they must have felt. They probably thought I was wallowing in self-pity. I had to appear incredibly selfish; that I couldn't get past my own sadness long enough to give them a happy experience. I hated myself for that. I considered not going to those events anymore. But what kind of friend would that make me? This was a no-win situation. To isolate myself from the experience meant I didn't care for these friends. To show up meant that at best, I would cry alone the whole way home, and at its worst, I would hide away and cry the entire time there. The days of setting my sadness aside and 'sucking it up' for a few hours were long gone. Infertility was a badge I wore on my heart with a button that could be pushed by anyone at any time.

Chapter 9

*It Wasn't What I Wanted, but
Maybe it Was What I Needed*

I t sounds like this has been a horrible experience that I
wouldn't wish to go through again. In fact, on a daily
basis, I do reconsider my choices to cycle and recycle, to
spend all of our savings and to put my body through this for
so many years. But truly and deeply, there is nothing that
would make me want to change this. I may not be
physically, financially, or emotionally stronger, but
spiritually, I have grown to find a peace within myself that
I am certain I would never have found had it not been for
this disease.

Infertility can definitely be the process of losing
oneself, but it can also be the process of finding oneself. It
can bring a person to their knees or it can make you stand a
bit straighter. Sometimes it can do both. Prior to this
experience I would have considered myself lost in a
number of ways. I was young and felt invincible. I didn't
just think I could have it all, in many ways I felt that I

145

deserved to have it all. There was a sense of entitlement that comes from things coming easily. I ignored my passions in lieu of plans. I sacrificed temperance for immediate gratification, often leaving me empty and regretful. These years of struggle have necessarily brought me to a place where I am able to be more introspective. What I have discovered makes the experience purposeful and important.

I have known the joy of being pregnant, if only for a short time. I was given a gift, and had it not been for our struggles to conceive, I may very well have been one of those women who views pregnancy as a difficult time of high hormonal changes and uncontrollable urges. I could have easily taken those weeks for granted and complained my way through to the end. Because of infertility, I cherished deeply each and every day of my pregnancy, not in hindsight like many others, but in each moment. I knew our baby was a miracle before he was ever conceived. I thanked God then, as I do now, for the gift of carrying him.

Infertility has forced me to discover patience within myself that I hadn't known prior. I spent much of my twenties wanting and striving, for nothing in particular and everything in general. Like many women my age, nothing I had was good enough, or lasted long enough, or happened quickly enough. Life was a race to be won; to be the first with the job, the car, the home, the husband, and the babies. Anything short of first place might as well have been last place. I was the first to meet my husband, but the last to be married. Because of this, I was angry and frustrated that Mike didn't propose sooner. The need to fulfill that ideal of marriage like my friends, took precedence over the longevity and commitment we had to each other.

Now, in my thirties and having dealt with infertility for these four and a half years, life has dealt me a path that requires the dissolution of plans and perfection. The timeline to success that was once so important is now moot. Clarity comes after time has passed and I am thankful today to have let go of the urgency to follow the original plans. I have learned to place my heart with the value of the goal instead of the need to be "on track" with everyone else.

The simplest aspects to our married life hold a different meaning since our experiences with infertility. Our vows are more important to me and the words we shared have taken on a relevance that I wasn't able to appreciate when we spoke them in our twenties. "I love you" is no longer the expected line inside of a Valentine's Day card; it is something that I feel in a deeper, more mature way. The person who once prided herself on being independent and not needing anyone exists only in vague shadows. Now not only do I need Mike, but I want to need him.

I know from my own life that it would be easy for people to see me and think, "She's got it made." My husband is the kindest and most generous man I could ever know. I have an amazing home filled with so many lovely material items. I am employed in a job that allows me to give of myself in a way that betters society, and explore my own creativity each day. In many ways I do have everything that a person could hope for. But I also have infertility. It is a weight that I carry physically and emotionally. It is because of this disease that I no longer see people for what they have, what they wear, or how they present themselves at face value. I no longer feel the envy of wanting to be someone else, because I understand that everyone has their own struggles that I may not be able to handle.

I am more aware of the pains of others. Where the words "get over it" or "suck it up" might have been a common phrase in my once tough exterior, I am now far

147

more empathetic to others. While it is natural for us to compare one person's issues to our own and chalk their problems up as trite in comparison, I understand, because of my infertility, a different perspective. It doesn't matter if I agree or disagree with their personal battles, everyone wants to be valued. They want their struggles to be felt by just one other person without judgment or being told how they should be handling it, or what they would do if they were in that position. Empathy is to identify with someone on the most human level and to find relevance in their situation.

Infertility does not make victims, it makes survivors. Even when I felt that my life was out of control and that I was sucked in cycle after cycle, I always knew Mike and I were the ones making the ultimate decisions on treatment. We were never at the mercy of doctors, technology or research. Even when there was no more money to pursue alternative avenues for conception, we had a wealth of power. Our faith in each other and the path we were on drove us to move forward each step of the way. We knew infertility was a part of our collective story, but it wasn't our whole story.

A word from Mike:

I believe that the most positive thing I have experienced from our infertility challenges is just how important a family is to us. Each time we received disappointing news, it just made us stronger and more determined. We would only allow a short amount of time of self-pity before planning our next move in our quest to have a family. Jenna would often say, "Okay, our five minutes are up, now what?" Granted, as the cycles evolved, five minutes became five days, but the point was noted and we moved forward together. When we finally are lucky to be blessed with a family, it will not go unappreciated.

Infertility has also taught me just how strong a person Jenna is. It amazes me every day to see what she has to go through. I honestly do not know if I could withstand all the tests and medicines she has taken. I also can't get over the medical knowledge she has gained over the past few years. I feel like my wife has morphed from a school teacher to research scientist to motivational speaker! Her determination through this whole process just fortifies my belief of how great of a mother she will be.

This experience made us increasingly aware of how important it was to follow a budget and prioritize our goals in life. As the medical bills swarmed the mailbox, it was crucial that we had some tough conversations about what was considered a "like to have" and a "need to have" item. We both traded in our cars to get junkers so we could increase our monthly cash flow. We also cut our food budget in half and went out only on special occasions. Although it felt like punishment at first, it quickly turned to a positive thing. We were both looking to our future.

I found that a lot of couples don't have the kind of communication that Jenna and I do. It's been because of our infertility that we have to sit together and make concrete decisions on a regular basis. Before this struggle, I played the finance role and Jenna took care of the house. It would have been easy for us to take each other's roles for granted. With days on bed rest and bills to pay, we have had to constantly help each other out and take an active role in the entire marriage, not just our established areas of comfort.

Being a mother is a calling that hasn't been realized yet. It isn't a dream or a desire. Winning the lottery, having a new wardrobe, or taking a trip around the world; those are dreams and desires. If they don't come true, life will go on. Disappointment comes from realizing a dream won't become a reality. But a calling is far different. It pushes me on when all rational thoughts are lost, and it makes it possible for me to scrape myself off the couch in the moments I'm paralyzed by sadness. This calling is what gets me to work each day and it feeds off the energy of the children I teach. Anyone who has felt a calling for anything can understand that there is no room for doubt. A calling doesn't let you doubt.

The day came where there were no more tests to run and there were no more protocols to invest in. We sat in our doctor's office and listened for the words that every infertile fears is an eventuality in their hearts. "There is really nothing different we can offer you." In those words the past years of anxiety, heartache, tears, happiness, excitement, fear, prayers and dreams culminated in the most vulnerable part of my being. I was only 31 years old when those words were spoken to me, and I felt I had aged 20 years.

My immediate reaction was to fight and continue fighting with every ounce of passion and determination I could find within myself. I knew that there were other tests and even though this, my second doctor, was at the bottom of her bag of tricks, there were others out there pioneering new procedures and testing new theories. I knew that this was not the end all and be all of our infertility.

For weeks I would visit message boards where kind and compassionate infertiles shared new protocols and medical journal articles to assist each other in the quest for that elusive baby to hold. In just a few days I had compiled a list of other treatments and experimental procedures. The list was long and overwhelming. In terms of what we had been through, this list redefined "struggle". One afternoon, I stepped away from my computer for some lunch. I found myself walking up the stairs to the second floor, and the next thing I knew, I was in the would-be nursery. I heard the words of my doctor echo in my heart, *There is really nothing different we can offer.* I felt a deep breath expand my lungs. A burning sensation filled my nostrils and I closed my eyes as tears fell down my cheeks.

Was it a death sentence? Strangely no. It was an answer; something we didn't have in all of the years of testing, monitoring and cycling. We had needed closure on our battle and it had come; not in the form a baby as we had hoped, but still, it was a moment of clarity.

I desire the experience of pregnancy. Strangely, I desire the morning sickness, fatigue, constipation and hemorrhoids to complain about. I desire a child with my husband's calm disposition and beautiful blue eyes. I desire a child who has my passionate opinions and determination that can often be misunderstood as stubbornness. I may not realize my desires, but life will go on. I will, however, realize my calling. I was meant to change this world with the institution of family. This is what I know to be true. I will be a mother. That may come when we have saved enough money to pursue adoption, or in time, when the wounds have healed, we may decide to continue on the path of IVF or any number of alternative treatments. 'How' and 'when' may be questionable, but 'if' is not a concern.

This story doesn't have a happily ever after. Not yet. Truthfully, I don't think that kind of ending belongs here anyway, and maybe that's why I was given this challenge of being infertile. Maybe I was meant to share with others that IVF isn't always the answer and that there's a lot more to infertility than just adopting or taking a vacation.

I haven't gotten to the pot of gold. This is the other side

of the rainbow; the part where everyone starts, where the end seems so far away, where the dreams and possibilities are infinitely distant. Yet, even at our darkest hours, the light at the end of the rainbow warms our hardened hearts and inspires all of us, no matter how remote we feel from it.

My frames remain empty today, but it will not be that way forever. They await, as I do, for the day when they will be displayed proudly on a wall in our upstairs hallway. They will tell a story not of pain, or of sadness, but of determination, and of love. Yes, today they are empty picture frames, but empty only of pictures, not of hope. Hope is the one thing they are filled with.

Chapter 10

~Post Script~
What to Do When You
Don't Know What to Do

H aving read this book, it must seem overwhelming to consider just how close infertility can come to consuming not only the individual, but all of the loved ones that want only the very best for him/her. In a valiant attempt to support those around us, many people on the fertile side of the world make some common missteps. In turn, the infertiles might often become angry and feel alone when all the fertile wanted to do was help.

I truly think infertile people are defensive about their disease because it has been so widely misunderstood. We live in a society which tends to view infertiles as pathetic and desperate, because we continued on this path without reward. Yet the same society seems to support women who had achieved success through the very same measures. They are deemed courageous and determined. What is the difference between us? Would the same people who tell us to move on dare to tell our successful counterparts that the children they conceived were a mistake and that they, too, should have moved on earlier? They had already won the war, and we are still in the battlefield.

I don't want to attack any of the fertiles out there, I just feel obligated to explain how and why your well-intentioned comments that are made out of love and support will naturally fall painfully on the heart of a person struggling to conceive. I've heard many of these suggestions myself, and from the closest people in my life. It is probably because they were so important to me that I held my friends and family to an impossible standard. I expected them to be in my head and to see the pain that, I thought, was written so plainly across my face.

1. **The story of the "person I know who was in your situation and it worked for them":**

I think it's part of the human experience to want to connect with those we love. We want to let them know they aren't alone and that there are others out there who have gone through this. The problem is, unless you were one of those people, the anecdote about the friend of a second cousin who had twins after her IVF isn't a story that's going to help. I know you are thinking this story shows empathy and will validate the infertile. However, the only thing your story will accomplish is to make an infertile feel more isolated. You see, if they are going through the process, it's because they *don't* have a baby, and to hear about someone so remotely related to you who succeeded means you couldn't think of anyone who truly is going through the pain that your friend is experiencing in that moment. Your second cousin's friend succeeded and while you think that will bring hope, it may only serve to prove that they are alone in their current failure. In an earlier section, I discussed how addicting treatments can be, but this is an appropriate time to also touch up on that topic.

During our early days of infertility, I used to hear stories all the time about the distant aunt, the neighbor and even the celebrity who went through six or more IVF cycles lasting years longer than I had experienced. Finally, their happy ending came when they discovered that they were pregnant, and with twins no less. HURRAY!!! "It can happen for you, too" is the customary follow up to the story. The problem was, these stories planted the seed in my mind that if I could just keep going, I would eventually find the success enjoyed by other people. These stories, although sometimes encouraging, were more often the very stories that stopped me from being able to mourn the lost cycles and accept the possibility of not mothering biological children. I thought I'd be giving up too soon, or that if I did give up on treatments, it meant I didn't want a child as badly as those that stuck it out and got their babies.

2. **"You are so stressed out about having a baby. Why don't you try to relax; go on a vacation, take a break from thinking about this."**

Again, you are probably thinking that this little goodie, whether in the form of an uplifting anecdote or a piece of advice, is just the kind of thing to make your infertile friend feel like there are miracles in the world and that she has as good a chance as anyone at being one of those. The problem is, many infertiles, like me, live in a perpetual state of fear, excitement, and crushing disappointment. To suggest that a vacation is going to fix their problems does nothing more than trivialize those feelings. Some of the people who make this recommendation do so because they heard a story of a family member who went on a tropical getaway and found themselves pregnant upon returning. It probably seemed like a miracle, but I'm willing to bet that the people they speak of did not suffer with infertility that was tested through numerous failures with the most extreme medical interventions. Some of them never even visited with a reproductive endocrinologist at all. Your infertile friend may have a structural abnormality that prevents an embryo from implanting, or is going through early menopause, or has never ovulated and/or menstruated in her entire life, or has a partner who is unable to produce sperm for any number of reasons. These are medical issues that aren't going to magically go away because they go on a vacation somewhere. Stress is caused by infertility, not the other way around. Then again, if you want to pay for a vacation to test your theory, I'm sure you won't be turned down.

3. **"I know someone who adopted after years of trying, and then they got pregnant on their own."**

First of all, adoption isn't a cure for infertility, no more so than a wig is a cure for cancer. It may help to heal one symptom of the disease, but it still needs to be a managed. It's absurd to compare adoption to infertility treatments on any level beyond the fact that they are both ways of building a family. I think any adopted child would be heartbroken to learn that they were brought into a family in the hopes that their parents would suddenly become pregnant from the process of adopting them. Secondly, this "miracle" of adoption ending years of true infertility is unfounded. Only a fractional percentage of couples find they are pregnant after beginning the adoption process. We don't know how many of those ever underwent extensive procedures versus those who tried naturally and then moved on to adoption prior to a diagnosis of "infertility". Sure, some people do get pregnant after adopting, just like some people walk away from a car crash without a seatbelt, but I wouldn't recommend that as a responsible practice.

As an aside to the adoption conversation, I think it's important to note that adoption is a lifetime commitment to a child. It is not a consolation prize for the loser of a game show. Children are a blessing, and adopted children are as much of a blessing to infertiles as they would be to fertile people. Yet many people assume that adoption is reserved only for those who cannot conceive naturally. If you are a fertile parent to biological children and have made a suggestion of adoption to someone who is working through infertility treatments, you should ask yourself why you didn't adopt. To this I would offer that adoption is not a process to be taken lightly. Just like preparing to have a biological child, having an adopted child requires an entirely new conversation and a serious personal evaluation. It is a marriage of sorts; a commitment to the life of another human being. Some couples, infertile or not, cannot make this assertion. For others, it takes a tremendous amount of love and planning.

When Mike and I were in the beginning steps of our treatments, there were several people who asked us, "Why don't you just adopt?" They said it as if we could just order a baby off a menu and pick it up at the drive-thru window. *Just adopt? And that's going to fix everything?* It's a ludicrous thought, not to mention highly offensive. Adoption wasn't going to cure our infertility or end my lifetime battle with amenorrhea. Each step in planning for a family, whether it was infertility treatments, various testing, or surrogacy, required intense conversations between Mike and me. None of those conversations were ever easy, and the most difficult was the one concerning adoption. It wasn't because either of us was opposed to being adoptive parents, in fact we both were excited about the prospect of realizing our parenting goals. It was difficult nevertheless because it meant opening ourselves up to an entirely new process that could be just as painful, just as rewarding, just as costly, and as stressful as the infertility we had been fighting for years. If it was as simple as "why don't you just adopt" I would have been first in line and I would have ordered a double.

4.   "Have you tried…?"

Chances are you don't need to finish that question. The answer is usually "yes". No infertile gets to be infertile unless they have been through a wringer of exams, read a half dozen books, and spent hours and hours researching on the internet, in medical journals, or in consultations with the best doctors their money can afford. They are experts on their bodies and are the first in line to consider every possible old wives tale before undergoing invasive medical treatments. I can tell you, as a veteran at the IVF thing, I had tried Robitussion, green tea, Mucinex, acupuncture, herbs, vitamins and supplements, chiropractic, exercise, yoga, meditation, and prayer. In addition to this, I've been tested for Celiac disease, I've had an MRI to look for tumors, we've undergone genetic testing on ourselves, as well as the baby I carried, I've been in stirrups more times than a jockey, eaten only warm foods, and I've spent $200 each week on an all organic diet, and a myriad of other treatments that I'd researched or heard about. If I was told that standing on my head and singing "Yankee Doodle" got someone pregnant, you can bet I would have given it a shot. It might sound pathetic and desperate, but many of these infertile loved ones are paying for their treatments with no help from insurance companies, so they will do anything to improve their chances. The point is, your well-intentioned suggestions might only frustrate a person who is doing everything in their power to succeed. I once had someone suggest to me that I should try ovulation predictor kits. With an initial diagnosis of anovulation, the inability to ovulate, this was little more than a slap in the face. We were three years into trying and had gone through two rounds of IUI and one IVF cycle when those words were shared with me. Their helpful suggestions only proved that they didn't know the first thing about what I was going through.

5. The power of "positive thinking".

I can't tell you how many people have suggested that I somehow created my reality with negative thoughts. The danger in this pearl of wisdom is that infertility immediately becomes my fault, something generated in my own psyche. Many infertiles already feel a sense of guilt and shame over their inability to perform the function that seems inherent in being a woman. Please don't further this notion by insisting that they can *think* their way out of it. Consider this: at the beginning of their long journey into infertility most women are filled with excitement. They are certain that it will all happen as it does in the movies; the husband, the home, the car, the pets, the children. There is not even the slightest consideration that they will not conceive that baby and live happily ever after. Essentially, there is not just positive thoughts running through their heart, but they nurture those loving emotions through each and every disappointing cycle. If positive thinking was what created a baby, there would be no infertility. Infertility isn't like wanting to find a soul mate or desiring a better job; it's a disease. We can control our attitude towards it, but we can't control the physical make-up of our bodies. Somewhere there must be action and intervention to support our efforts.

6. "Be grateful for what you do have," aka "Things could be worse."

Of course it could be. I could have a terminal illness. I could have every member of my family wiped away in a natural disaster. I could lose my job, my house, and my car all in the same day. My husband could leave me for another woman or man, or both! I've seen Jerry Springer. I know things could always be worse. Everyone is given what they can handle and they either rise to the moment or fall forlornly to a pit of despair. Please, I beg of you, do not share with your infertile friend how their life could be worse. Chances are they think about this all the time as if waiting for the other shoe to fall. The saying 'misery loves company' does not apply to this situation.

I had one person tell me that I needed to be more grateful for what life brought me and focus on what I do have, as if to suggest that I was selfishly wanting more and more and never taking the time to appreciate what I have been fortunate for. This person used herself as an example. She said, "I've been through some hard times too, but I always remember that I have my husband and four children to bring me joy. Think about what you have." *Seriously? Are you kidding?* I wonder if she ever realized how effectively she disproved her own point by mentioning that it was her FOUR children that made her grateful for her life.

Another person relayed the story of her friend who had lost her leg from a debilitating disease and how she, herself, had dealt with muscular dystrophy for the better part of five years. When her story began, I actually thought that she was going to be someone with whom I was going to share compassion and that we'd be able to talk about how we're both better in many ways for the experience. Wrong! This person finished talking about her disease and then, like a slap in the face added, "So see, Jenna, be glad if not ever having a baby is *all* you have to deal with."

Minimizing someone's experiences is no way to be a good friend. Everyone has a story to share and a struggle that, to them, feels like the most they can possibly handle. Telling them that their issue is essentially not that big of a deal, whether it's a terrible cold, infertility, or a terminal illness, isn't a way to make them feel validated or empowered. It only makes them feel powerless.

7. Don't use the "Look on the bright side" approach.

One of the oddest responses to our infertility that I've received was when someone decided to explain all of the things Mike and I could do if we never had kids. In hindsight, I think this person probably felt very awkward about the seriousness of the topic and was trying to make it seem lighthearted. They made comments such as, "Enjoy your freedom while you have it", "Think about all the places you could go without kids", "You'll never have to worry about college tuition" and, "You'll be able to sleep in without worrying about kids to take care of" and the list could go on. The only thing I can equate this to would be to suggest that if your house burned down, and someone said to you, "Well at least you won't have to worry about a heating bill" or if you lost a loved one and someone said, "Think of the money you'll save on birthday presents." OUCH! You'd be thinking that the 'benefit' couldn't possibly compensate for the loss. You're right. That's how an infertile will perceive the same well-intentioned 'pep talk'.

I know, it sounds like there is nothing you can do that will be right. You might be thinking, "Do I have to walk on eggshells all the time?" Of course not. As important as it is to know what to avoid, there are so many things that you can do to truly help your infertile friend. Without realizing it, you aren't helpless to do something for the person you care for. In fact, you have more power than you could possibly realize. I remember my mother telling me that she would wake up in the middle of the night in a panic attack because there was nothing she could do. This is simply NOT true, but it's a common misconception.

Mike and I had taped the segment for the Oprah Winfrey Show on Halloween. Between October 31st and January 25th when it aired, we may have shared our impending appearance with a handful of friends and family. We were nervous about sharing our story with millions of viewers when we hadn't shared it with more than a dozen people prior. I was afraid of looking pathetic, of having my words twisted around, and mostly of being misunderstood by the people closest to me. The people that we chose to share our news with also knew that I was immensely self-conscious of the situation.

In the days that preceded the airing, I was filled with trepidation. I wasn't sure if the infertile community would see my segment as yet another step backwards, or if the people in my life would feel embarrassed by what I said and shared. Another part of me was ready to have it all on the table and end this secret for good. With an audience of millions, I felt that this was the ultimate "outing" and from that point on, people would know that I was ready to share my experiences and handle any questions. I was anxious to just be able to talk about it openly. I didn't know what to expect, but I definitely didn't expect what I got.

Nothing. Our house wasn't flooded with calls from family members or friends as I had thought. In the days that followed, I went to school and was stunned by the vast number of people who had seen the show and not spoken a word to me. It was like it never happened. Everywhere I went, whether it was to work or out with friends, it was as if they wanted my secret to remain just that. I began to feel that they were more comfortable avoiding the topic than addressing the elephant in the room. Thousands of people all over the internet had responded on message boards and other websites, and yet, here, in my small town, it was recognized by a total of four people; two of which I had never even met. Dozens of options ran through my mind. *Did I do horribly? Was the topic too embarrassing for people to handle? Did I look bad? Were they mad that I hadn't announced my appearance? What should I have done differently?*

Our family, friends and colleagues aren't bad people. They are, in fact, some of the most amazing individuals anyone could know. They weren't intentionally being insensitive, but in the days that followed our segment, I felt like the village pariah. The problem wasn't me and my over sensitivity, nor was it the people who loved me and what I then perceived as their lack of concern or uncertainty as to how to respond. No one was at fault, because no one caused the disease that was robbing us of our ability to conceive a baby. No, the problem, and the only true place to lay blame, was the disease, a disease where no one wins and there is no "right" way to act or react.

163

I know you don't know what to say or do, which is why so many people make all the mistakes listed above, or worse, they do what was done to me; avoid the topic completely for fear that they will say something offensive. Here are some things you could do during an incredibly difficult situation.

1. When they talk, listen.

One common misconception is that the infertile has no idea what they are doing wrong and they are looking for someone in the fertile world to review and correct their actions. On the contrary, the infertile isn't looking for advice. That is what their reproductive endocrinologist is for. In fact, if they are anything like me, they are pretty much topped off with advice. They've been hearing what they could do and what they should do from everyone on the internet and a half dozen second, third and fourth opinions. Doctors and specialists in all shapes and sizes spend hours talking at them. The infertiles listen, ask questions and get talked at some more.

What they are looking for from you is simply a sympathetic ear. They may be devastated by a recent failed cycle, and worried about the financial toll their cycles are taking on their retirements and savings. Sometimes they might need a shoulder to cry on when they feel like no one can understand how they feel. They might be anxious about a pregnancy test that is upcoming, or frustrated by the amount of information they've had to sift through regarding their condition. They might be moody from the intense hormone fluctuations, or feel exhausted by the constant poking and prodding of ultrasounds and blood work. Whatever it is, listen intently. Sometimes that is the best medicine your infertile friend needs.

2. When they don't talk, ask.

If you know about your friend's struggles, it is because they have trusted you with one of the most important and private aspects in their life. Don't forget that, and don't take it lightly. They may not talk about it all the time, and that's probably because infertility can feel like a tremendous burden; a burden they don't want you to carry, too. This doesn't mean they don't want to talk about it, it just means they are waiting for you to show interest. The way to do this is to ask anything and everything. If you don't understand a treatment, ask about it. Chances are the infertile will have a wealth of knowledge to share, and will welcome the chance to release some of the anxiety. Your questions show genuine interest and concern.

For some people it took weeks following the Oprah Show, to call or stop by to finally check in. By the time I was approached, I was clearly upset and carried a pretty decent sized chip on my shoulder because I felt so blatantly ignored when the show aired. Noticing my obvious frustration, some of these people defended their behavior by explaining that they didn't think I wanted to talk about it and were trying to give me some privacy. They thought I wanted space. *Space? The cavity I had felt between myself and the rest of the normal fertile world could have housed enough food to feed a third world country. Why on earth would I desire more space?* And to assume what I wanted? Why not just ask? Why not let me decide how I wanted to respond? To this, the response was something to the effect of, "You've always been very private about the situation." *For God's sake people, I put myself on national television. Any thoughts of privacy pretty much went out the window after that, don't you think?* Still, I can appreciate their truly sincere attempt at sensitivity. I can see where these people were coming from. They wanted to do the right thing, and certainly weren't intentionally disregarding the pain I felt. If they knew how I was feeling, I know they would have acted differently. As I said, this disease doesn't leave a lot of room for misunderstandings and miscommunication. Communication is the bridge between an isolated infertile and a confused friend.

Of course, there will be times when your infertile friend won't want to talk about it or share the dirty details. They might be at the end of a cycle and the anxiety is too much to talk about without crying. Or they might have received some disappointing news and needs time to digest it and grieve for a lost cycle. If that's the case, don't give up, but take a more subtle approach. Check in a day later, or write her a card just to let her know you are thinking of her. She'll need the support, and she'll be grateful that you are interested. Whatever you do, don't ignore her because you feel like you don't know what to say. She probably already feels alone, and pretending nothing is wrong might be a defense for feelings of helplessness. If your infertile loved one has been through the wringer of treatments, then they have probably also been through the gamut of bad experiences with outsiders. This will make them hesitant to share. Their defenses will be up and they might not want to put themselves in a position to be criticized for their efforts. If this is the case, they will need your support more than anything. They will need your interest and admiration for their efforts.

Thursday, July 28, 2005

Admittance into the Drug Store

Kerry and Trisha just left a little while ago. The boys are

playing poker tonight, so we decided to get some dinner and hang out over here. It was nice to have a night of friends and relaxation. It had been a while since the three of us hung out together. What was a simple night with friends turned into Jenna the Side Show.

Around 8:00 I had to go upstairs to do one of my injections. Trisha asked if she could help, but I told her I really didn't need any help. I could sense that what she was really asking was if she could come along and be a part of it. I offered for her to come and see the whole thing. I think that might have made it weird for Kerry, so she came as well. Up until tonight, I knew Kerry was aware of our problem having kids, but we hadn't really talked about it. Even with Trisha, my own sister, the conversations about infertility were brief. Having babies of their own makes them distant from infertility and the process is just too technical to really explain with any amount of justice.

The whole thing that usually takes a few minutes turned into a ten-minute lesson of each drug, needle, and the process in general. I could tell they were overwhelmed and intimidated by everything on the counter. That made me feel validated. I think the months of giving myself injections has made me sort of numb to the process. We hide away the pharmacy in our bathroom and up until tonight, no one has seen it but Mike and me.

Trisha said, "I'm amazed at how you do this every day." Wow! That was a great compliment, although I think it was probably more of an observation. I had felt really embarrassed that I couldn't have kids, and to know that someone saw me as strong for being able to keep the pace with it, was a good feeling.

Kerry said something about how she wouldn't be able to inject herself with those needles all the time. That was kind of funny. She said it like it was a choice. It's not like this is an option for me. Having a child might be a choice for some people, but having infertility immediately negates that choice. I said, "If you were told that this is what it took for you to have had your daughter, I don't think you would have hesitated. You'd be shocked what you can do when you need to."

As personal as the whole thing is, I know it makes them feel closer to me and to be honest, it was refreshing to have someone want to be a part of this. The ten minutes of awkwardness in the bathroom was worth it. Knowing that they can conceptualize this process hopefully will give them a better understanding of the emotions that go with everything. I don't know if it will lead to any more conversations about the whole thing, but it was a step forward for me to be able to talk about it..

3. Research.

Depending on how much you know about your loved one's situation, doing some research will most likely help. I just said that you should ask questions, but that is only true when the questions are relevant to what process she is experiencing. If your infertile friend is just starting out, it's probably not a good idea to throw around acronyms like "PGD", "GIFT", "IVF", "ZIFT" or "ICSI" just because you looked them up online. This is no time to flaunt your ability to surf the net. This will feel overwhelming and make a worrisome situation worse. Conversely, I was surprised at how many people I would talk to who had no idea how a baby was conceived, nor the internal structure of the female body. As I was trying to answer questions about exactly what the medications did to my body, I often found myself trying to create models with my arms and fingers of the uterus, fallopian tubes and ovaries. Being knowledgeable about the basic parts of the male and female reproductive systems is a first step that anyone can, and should, take. It's hard to have a conversation about infertility with someone who doesn't know the first thing about reproduction.

4. Help lighten the load.

One of the biggest strains of infertility treatments is the constant attention it demands. Patients undergoing treatment are actively involved in their cycles. It's not just a few doctor's appointments and then a baby is made in a Petri dish somewhere. During my sixth IVF cycle, I was taking nine different medications, four of which were injections that my husband and I would have to deliver to various parts of my body at specific times of the day or night. This was in conjunction with the regular appointments for blood draw and transvaginal ultrasounds before I ever made my way to school in the morning.

If you can do anything to help your loved one through a cycle, PLEASE do it. This could be anything from getting them a decaffeinated coffee in the morning, to helping them with their responsibilities at work. Sometimes even the simplest tasks can feel overwhelming in the middle of a medicated cycle.

I had a couple of wonderful friends who would cover my homeroom each morning that I was being monitored, and corrected writing projects for me so that I didn't have to feel anxious about my cycle affecting my students. My mother made me frozen dinners for my days of bed rest, and my husband made sure the house was always clean so that my Type A personality didn't stress out about the hair that accumulated in the shower drain. Anything you can do to ease the treatment cycle of an infertile won't fall deafly on her. It may not be immediately recognized, but I can tell you from experience that I have a lot of unborn children who are already named after the guardian angels who helped me along the way!

5. Be sensitive when it comes to pregnancy announcements, birthdays, Mother's Day, baby showers, and all other holidays.

What was once a reason to celebrate becomes a time of reflection for the infertile. Wounds that might have been on the road to recovery will open up immediately when a holiday or other such event rolls around. As you are off opening presents at a shower, or enjoying your Mother's/Father's day breakfast in bed, the infertile is alone and painfully aware of that fact. Chances are, they are feeling the polar opposite emotion that you are, but on the same level. Think of the strength of the happiness and joy you feel at a birthday party or pregnancy announcement for example. That is the same strength with which the infertiles are feeling isolated.

In saying this, I want to be careful that I don't give fertiles the impression that they should ignore their infertile counterparts when it comes to invitations to these kinds of events. Just the opposite is true. To avoid the invitation or announcement only serves to alienate the infertile more. So where's the middle ground? This is where the sensitivity comes into play. It may feel like she is pushing you away when she doesn't attend an event, but please don't be offended, and furthermore, please don't make her feel guilty by saying things like, "I'm disappointed that you won't be there." Instead, try something like, "I understand why that would be hard, but know I'll be thinking of you." No matter how close your relationship is, the vulnerability that comes from attending an event like a baby shower or birthday party often takes precedence.

In the beginning of my infertility battle, I was able to face these events with grace, but with time and failed cycles behind me, it became increasingly more difficult to

170

approach the same activities with enthusiasm. Trust your infertile friend to know her limits and respect the times when she isn't able to fulfill the social obligations.

6. Understand that loss is a universal emotion.

To make this easier to understand I would offer that you think about infertility in the same light as you would any other loss. Whether it be the death of a pet, relative, or friend, the pain of that loss will eventually lessen, but will never entirely go away. You wouldn't wake up one day thinking about a lost grandparent and say, "Oh that doesn't bother me anymore. I'm over it." Infertility and miscarriage are losses on a different level. There is no statue of limitation for grieving

Time may make things better in some ways, but the wound of miscarriage and infertility is something that I am certain to bear for the remainder of my days. Yet, this kind of loss is always a source of tremendous misunderstanding for my fertile counterparts. I beg of each and every friend or loved one to do as much research as you possibly can when miscarriage and infertility finds a home in your circle of acquaintances. At a time of grief and emptiness, the hardest part for me was trying to find the words to express my sadness. Many times I felt compelled to justify why I was still upset over the loss of our son. For many people he was too abstract to comprehend.

Allow empathy to be your guide on this one. Each person experiencing miscarriage or infertility will deal with their circumstances differently. Some will seek professional counseling, while others will depend on the patience of friends. Still others will feel the need to jump back on the horse and try again. Mostly, I would offer that long after you have forgotten, and moved on with the rigors of life, the element of miscarriage and infertility will continue to surface time and time again. Birthday parties, camping trips, diaper commercials, and the "baby" section of the greeting card aisle may be the spoon that stirs the pot of emotions. Our experiences with infertility and miscarriage are something we will get through, but we may not get over.

7. Whatever you do, remember infertility is a disease.

This is probably the most important suggestion I can offer. If you've had the misfortune to know anyone with any kind of disease, possibly yourself, then you know that the extent to which it can affect your life will range from the type and stage of the disease, to the person who is dealing with it. But one thing is constant. It is an affliction that will always be a part of the person's past, present and in many ways, they will carry it into the future, regardless of the outcome. The American Society for Reproductive Medicine (ASRM) recognizes infertility as a disease. If you can think of it that way, you'll be less likely to make the mistakes of trivializing the experience. Would you tell an alcoholic to have a drink and relax? Would you tell someone with high cholesterol to simply "let it go?" Would you tell a friend suffering from the debilitating effects of ALS to think positively and take a vacation? I should hope not. We are compassionate to those who are fighting a disease and we admire their ability to face it with dignity and courage. Why is infertility different? Is it because you can't see anything on the surface to distinguish them from healthy people? Look again. The infertile's arms may be covered in small bruises from the needles used to draw their blood every other day, or look around their belly

172

button and see the tiny pin holes where they've injected their daily doses of medication, or the heavy knots on their rear ends where the injections of progesterone in oil have coagulated, making it difficult to sit down comfortably. But perhaps the hardest mark to miss is the sadness that is often clearly displayed on their face, but is covered in vain with the daily functioning of life. The marks are there, and they are a painful reminder of a disease that is, in many ways, incapacitating.

When all else fails~

Some of the kindest words I ever heard were from someone who said, "I don't know what to do for you." And then she followed it up with, "I can't imagine what you are going through." Finally! Someone who was honest and could look at our situation without the need or desire to fix what was seemingly unfixable in the end. It was refreshing to have someone else be able to admit defeat in the face of such an antagonist. The person who spoke those words won me over and began a crack in a fairly bitter shell. It was one of the few times when I felt like someone validated my experience and took the time to come down to where I was at emotionally.

An amazing thing happened. From a place of sorrow and shame, I felt strong again. It was remarkable that this person who didn't "know what to do" did exactly the right thing. She didn't judge my situation, or make claims on how to fix it, or try to cheer me up, or change the subject to something more pleasant. She made me feel like I could open myself up to the possibility that perhaps I wasn't alone or misunderstood. When all else fails, or maybe before anything has failed, facing ignorance can be the most sensitive thing to do.

Glossary of Terminology

andrologist: A physician-scientist who performs clinical or laboratory evaluations of male fertility.

anovulation: absence of ovulation when it would normally be expected.

assisted reproductive technology: All treatments that include the handling of eggs and/or embryos, such as in vitro fertilization (IVF).

basal body temperature (BBT): By carefully measuring BBT every morning before getting out of bed and recording it on a chart, many women are able to estimate when they are ovulating. This helps pinpoint when a woman is most and least likely to become pregnant. The thermometer used for measuring the BBT is marked in tenths of a degree, making it possible to detect even small rises in temperature. When the temperature goes up-usually about 0.4°F (0.2°C) to 1.0°F (0.6°C)-and stays up for several days in a row, ovulation has occurred.

body mass index (BMI): BMI is a simple mathematical formula, based on height and weight, that is used to measure content.

Clomiphene citrate (Clomid): stimulates the release of hormones that trigger ovulation. Clomiphene is typically the first choice of treatment for unexplained lack of ovulation. Due to its ease of use-it's taken orally rather than injected—it doesn't usually cause severe side effects, and doesn't usually require daily monitoring.

dilation and evacuation (D&E): a process in which the cervix is dilated and the uterus is cleaned. Today D&C's are often performed using suction (as opposed to the more aggressive method of scraping the uterus). One of the main reasons a D&E is performed is when excess tissue needs to be removed from the uterus, e.g., after an incomplete miscarriage where not all the tissue associated with the pregnancy was expelled naturally.

egg retrieval: A procedure to obtain eggs from the ovarian follicles. The procedure is performed using a needle and ultrasound to locate the follicle in the ovary.

embryo: A fertilized egg that has begun cell division.

embryo transfer: Placing an egg fertilized outside the womb into a woman's uterus.

embryologist: one who studies the development of an embryo.

frozen embryo transfer (FET): The transfer to the uterus of remaining embryos resulting from IVF / ICSI that were frozen for future use.

gamete intrafallopian transfer (GIFT): involves collecting eggs from the ovaries, then placing them into a thin flexible tube with the sperm. This is then injected into the woman's fallopian tubes where fertilization takes place.

human chorionic gonadotropin (hCG): is sold under many brand names. This hormone stimulates the gonads in both men and women. In men, hCG increases androgen production. In women, it increases the levels of progesterone. Human chorionic gonadotropin can help stimulate ovulation in women.

hyperstimulation: A condition caused by overstimulation of the ovaries that may cause painful swelling of the ovaries and fluid in the abdomen and lungs.

hypothalamic amenorrhea: The term hypothalamic refers to the hypothalamus, an area at the base of the brain that acts as a hormone control center for the body, regulating, among other things, a woman's menstrual cycle. In certain situations, such as anorexia, excessive exercise and stress, the flow of hormones is interrupted. This results in the failure of the body to produce enough estrogen and progesterone, the suppression of ovulation, and ultimately, the loss of menses.

hysterosalpingogram: an X-ray test that examines the inside of uterus and fallopian tubes.

hysteroscopy: a diagnostic and surgical procedure that makes examining the inside of the uterus possible without making an abdominal cut (incision). During hysteroscopy, a lighted viewing instrument called a hysteroscope is inserted through the vagina and cervix and into the uterus. Treatment can also be done through the hysteroscope during the same procedure.

intracytoplasmic sperm injection (ICSI): the injection of a single sperm into an egg. The fertilized egg is then placed in the woman's uterus or fallopian tube. Used with in vitro fertilization, ICSI is often a successful treatment for men with impaired sperm.

intrauterine Insemination (IUI): This procedure is often combined with hormone treatments to boost egg production. It can help couples with low sperm count, mild endometriosis, or cervical mucus problems. Semen is collected then delivered via a catheter inserted through the women's vagina and cervix to her uterus.

in vitro fertilization: May help those with pelvic or tubal damage, or male infertility. The woman takes drugs to stimulate egg production, and then eggs and sperm (from her partner or a donor) are collected, combined, and inserted into her body to develop. "In vitro" means "in glass" (that is, in a test tube or laboratory dish).

pre-genetic diagnosis (PGD): A procedure performed in conjunction with IVF in which one or two cells are removed from an embryo prior to the initiation of pregnancy and screened for genetic abnormalities.

Provera: Medroxyprogesterone is used to treat abnormal menstruation (periods) or irregular vaginal bleeding. Medroxyprogesterone is also used to bring on a normal menstrual cycle in women who menstruated normally in the past, but have not menstruated for at least six months, and who are not pregnant or undergoing menopause (change of life). Medroxyprogesterone is also used to prevent overgrowth of the lining of the uterus (womb) and may decrease the risk of cancer of the uterus in patients who are taking estrogen. Medroxyprogesterone is in a class of medications called progestins. It works by stopping the growth of the lining of the uterus and by causing the uterus to produce certain hormones.

reproductive endocrinologist: Reproductive endocrinologists are medical doctors who specialize in the care and treatment of women who have trouble becoming pregnant or who have other reproductive or hormonal disorders.
Reproductive endocrinologists are gynecologists who specialize in infertility. They can be board-certified through the Board of Obstetrics and Gynecology, which is recognized by the American Board of Medical Specialties.

surrogacy: In traditional surrogacy, another woman carries and gives birth to a baby conceived with her egg and the partner's sperm (through artificial insemination). In gestational surrogacy, the surrogate carries and gives birth to a baby conceived with the patient's egg and her partner's sperm, then transferred as an embryo to the surrogate's womb.

transvaginal ultrasound: Ultrasound imaging of the female reproductive system through an ultrasound device inserted into the vagina.

zygote intrafallopian transfer (ZIFT): combines IVF and GIFT. Eggs and sperm are mixed outside of the body. The fertilized eggs (zygotes) are then returned to the fallopian tubes, through which they travel to the uterus.

Acknowledgments

"Gambler's_fallacy." *Wikipedia, the free encyclopedia.* 02 Mar. 2007. <Reference.com http://www.reference.com/browse/wiki/Gambler's_fallacy>

Kubler-Ross, E (2005) *On Grief and Grieving: Finding the Meaning of Grief Through the Five Stages of Loss,* Simon & Schuster Ltd.

"Fast Facts about Infertility." Resolve. RESOLVE: The National Infertility Association. 10 Mar 2007 <http://www.resolve.org>.

"ART 2004 Home Page." Center for Disease Control and Prevention. 08 Feb 2007. Department of Health and Human Services. 10 Mar 2007 <http://cdc.gov>.

"Frequently Asked Questions About Infertility." American Society for Reproductive Medicine. 2007. American Society of Reproductive Medicine. 10 Mar 2007 <http//www.asrm.org>.

Cooke, Kerry, and Fackler, Amy. "Assisted Reproductive Technology." <u>Healthwise</u> (2006) <http://www.webmd.com>.

Printed in the United States
112621LV00002B/57/A

9 781432 705961